DATE DUE

~~AP 19 '96~~		
~~FE 12 '98~~		
~~MR 16 '98~~		
~~NO 20 '99~~		

DEMCO 38-296

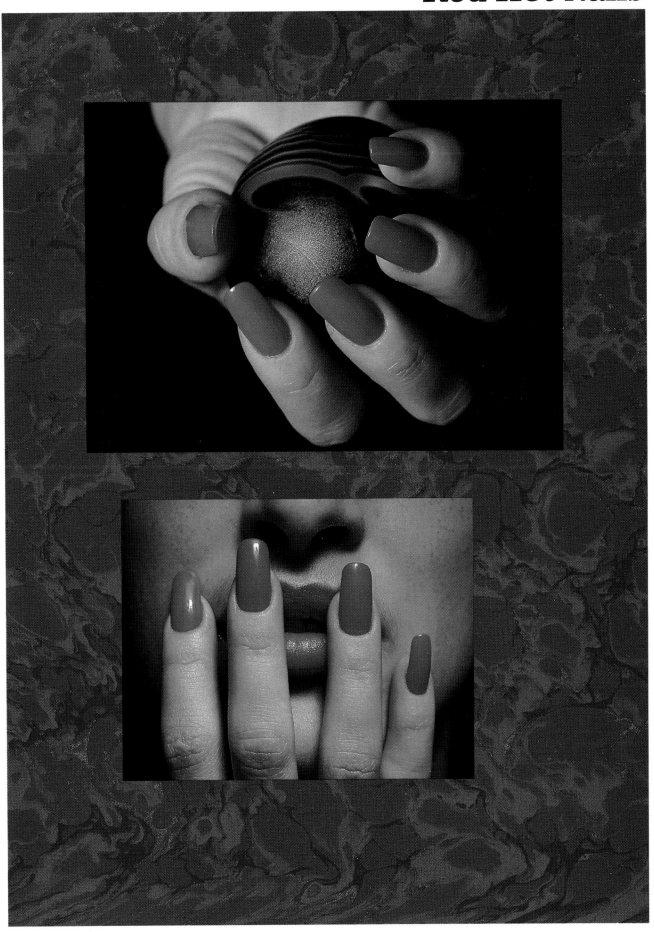

Diamonds are a Girl's Best Friend

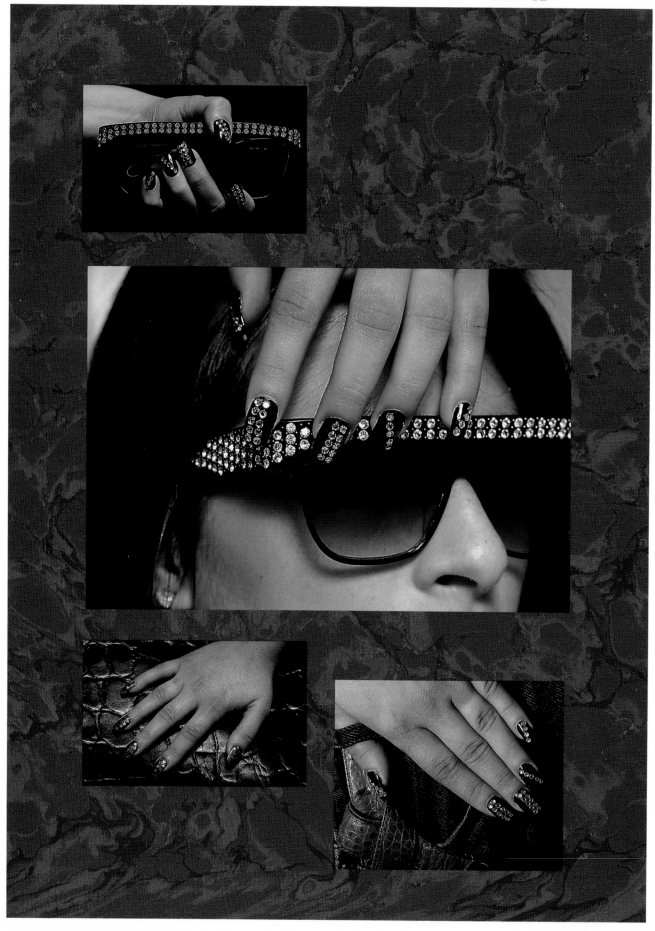

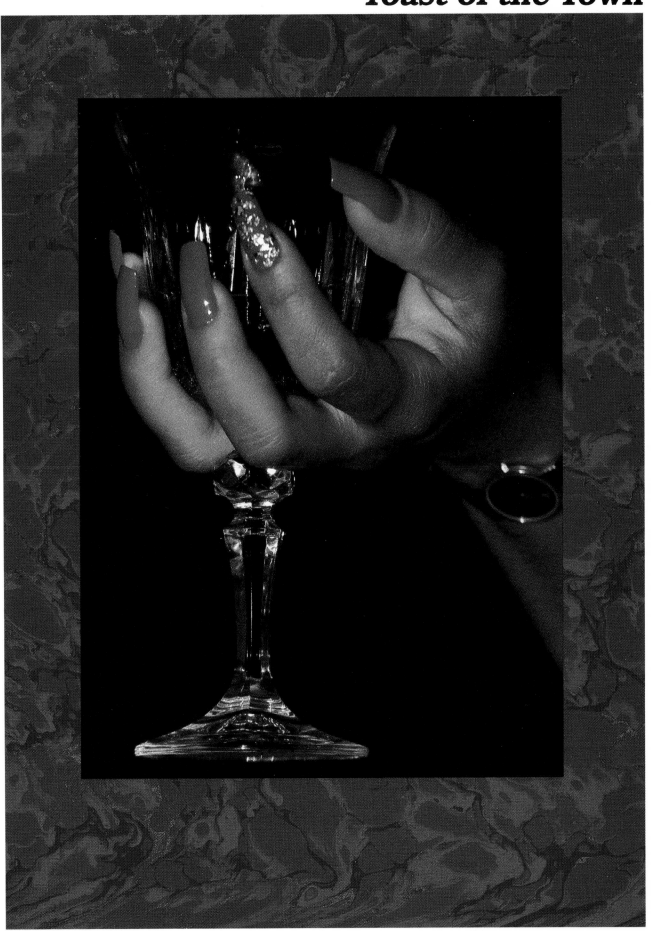

Simply Sensational

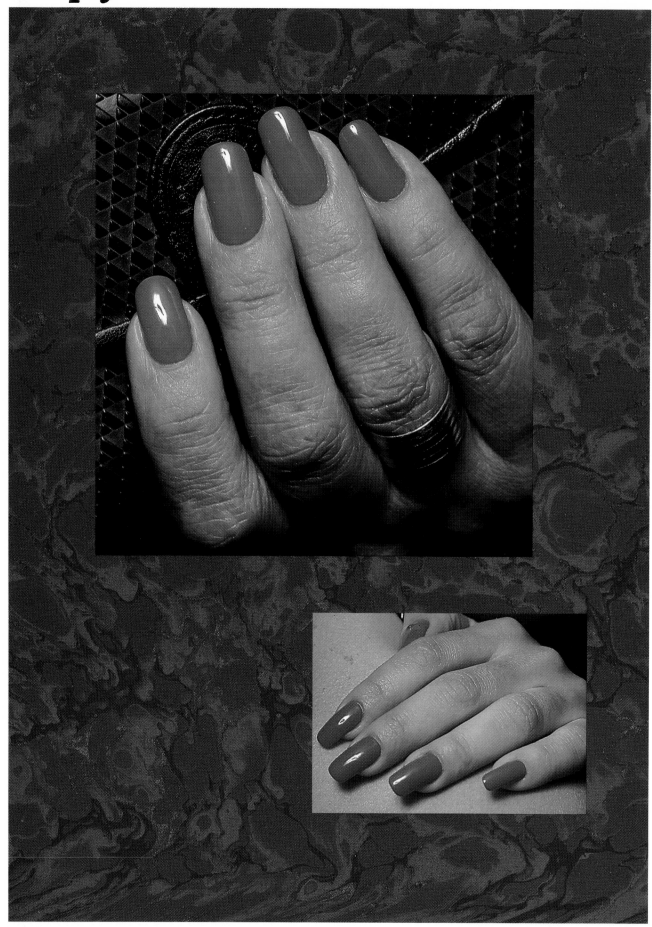

Adding Sparkle with Gold Leaf and Rhinestones!

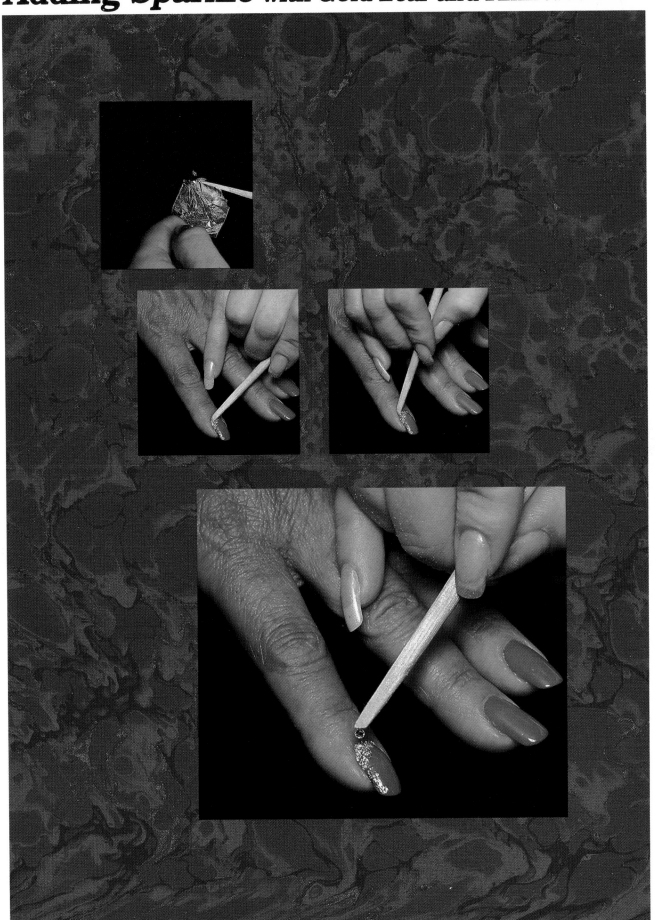

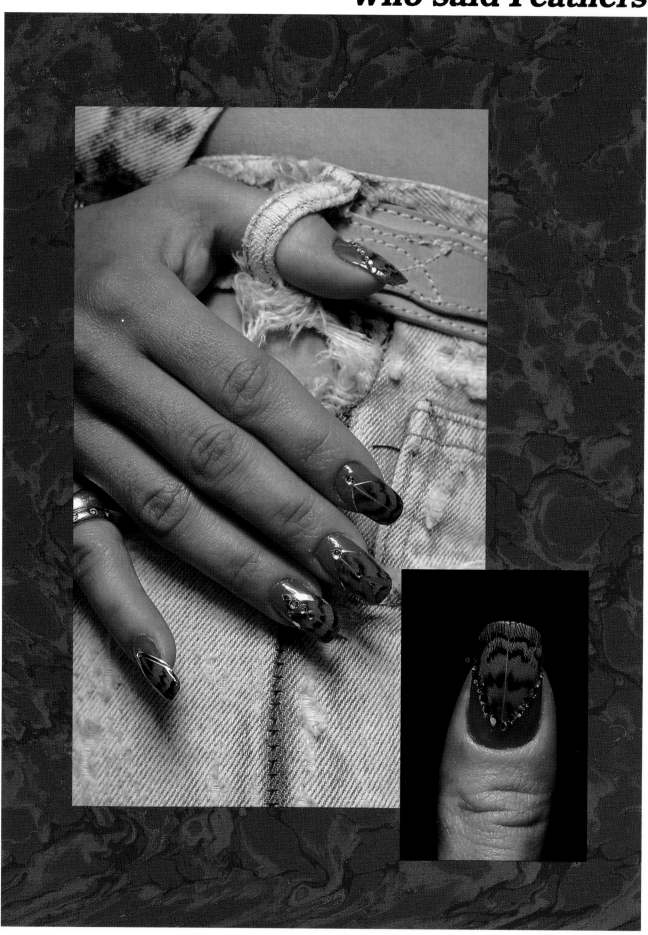

were out of Vogue?

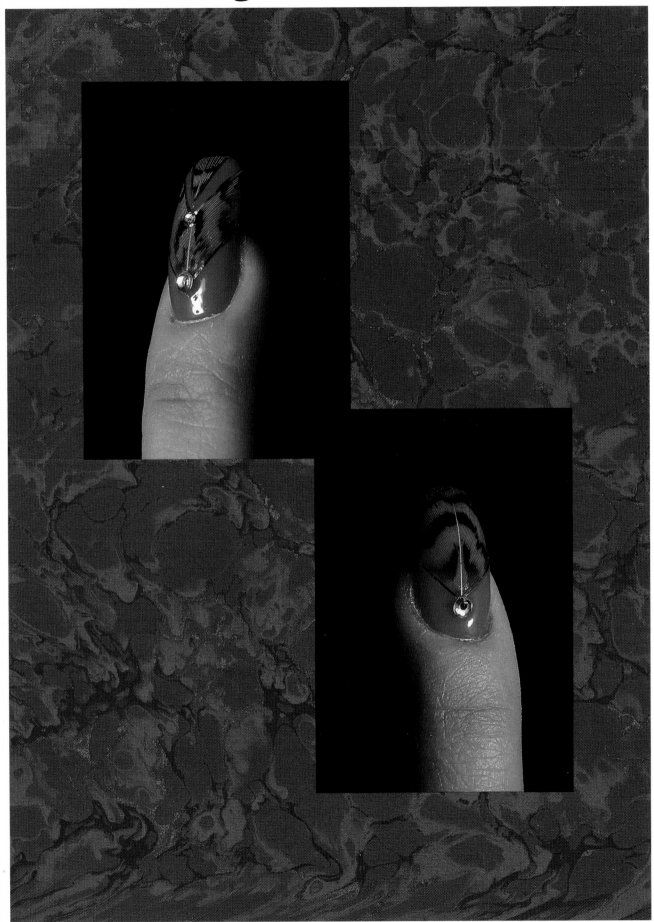

Purely Parisian — The French Manicure

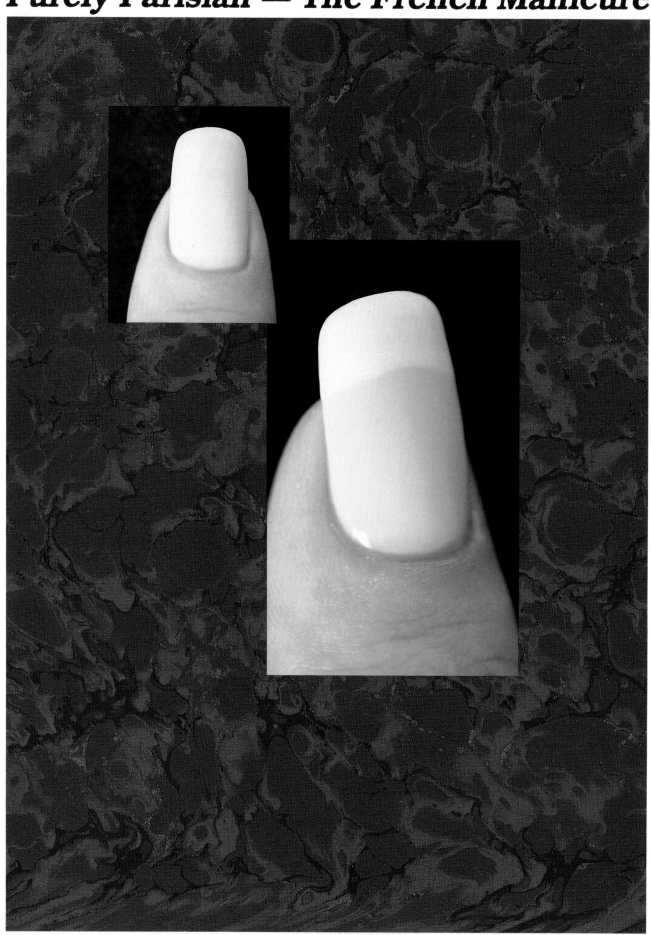

techNAILS

techNAILS

Extensions, Wraps, and Nail Art

Tammy Bigan

Milady Publishing Company
(A Division of Delmar Publishers Inc.)
3 Columbia Circle Drive
Albany, NY 12212

Editor:	Catherine Frangie
Editorial Assistant:	Jaqueline Flynn
Production Manager:	John Mickelbank
Art Coordinator:	John Fornieri
Photographer:	Howard Wechsler
Cover Artist:	Raymond Morelli

Copyright © 1992
Milady Publishing Company
(A Division of Delmar Publishers Inc.)

Printed in the United States of America

10 9 8 7 6 5 4 3

ISBN 0-87350-382-1

Library of Congress Cataloging-in-Publication Data

Bigan, Tammy.
    Technails / by Tammy Bigan.
        p.   cm.
    ISBN 0-87350-382-1 :
      1. Nails (Anatomy)—Care and hygiene.   2. Fingernails—Care and
  hygiene. 3. Manicuring. I. Title.
  RL94.B54 1992   91-8709
  646.7'27—dc20   CIP

Dedication

To all people who want to learn a way to become self-sufficient, creative, and giving, I dedicate this book.

Tammy Bigan

With Special Thanks

To my husband Andrew for supporting all my efforts in getting this project done.

To Diana A. Correa for typing this book for me, helping me put it all together, and for hanging in to the end.

To Danton Thompson who said, "Why don't you write a book!"

To Dale Bona, Betty Romesburg, and Anne Fretto for reviewing *techNAILS* and for their helpful suggestions.

Contents

Foreword

The nail care business has never been better. It can be a great profession that is self and financially rewarding. It is great to make people feel better about themselves, knowing that long after they leave you, they will look at their hands and see how beautiful you made them. On the other hand, the potential profits can be endless depending on your knowledge of the trade. You can start doing nails on a part-time basis while gaining experience and developing your technique. Eventually, you could have your own nail salon. In addition, selling nail products is very profitable as well as a service to clients. Recognition and respect for nail technicians is growing. Let's keep it going by keeping our standards high.

Proper training in procedure and development of technique is important in being successful. Knowing the proper use of supplies is very important in achieving desired results. Improper use can be harmful. Easy to follow instructions are designed for the beginner or for the existing professionals who need to learn new techniques and supplies/products used. Practice will gain the most desired results in nail care.

Introduction

Advanced nail techniques allow almost anyone with undesirable nails to have beautiful nails thanks to the many ways to lengthen, strengthen, and shape them to perfection. All wrapping techniques add strength to natural nails, and protect them from daily wear and tear that might otherwise destroy them. If nails are short, they can be strengthened and lengthened by gluing a tip extension or making a sculptured nail with acrylic. No matter what type of extension is used, the main objective is to have natural nails with the aid of a wrap to keep it there. Extensions are eventually filed away during maintenance manicures and fill-ins. As the nail grows forward, the wrap and the extension move forward with it and the nail gets longer. To maintain a desired length, the nail must be shortened, thus removing one while replacing the other end which is the base of the nail. Little by little the extension is filed away and the natural nail is left under the wrap. This must be explained to every client receiving any type of wrap with an extension. When the natural nail gets to the desired length, the wrap is still needed. It would have never gotten so long without the wrap and it can't survive without it.

If a client has strong nails that don't need the wrap, but one nail breaks and the client wants an extension until it grows back, then only do maintenance manicures and file the extension a little each time.

No matter what wrapping or extending technique is being used, you must remember that the way you shape the nail with your file determines the end result.

Always try to preserve the natural nail and avoid damage by using great care in protecting it.

Take pride in your work and do the best you can.

Introduction to Advanced Nail Techniques

Nail care has been around for centuries. Once only a few could indulge in the luxury. Now, more people, both male and female, are getting their hands and feet cared for on a regular basis along with their hair and body. Nail care is included in total personal care.

The number of nail care services has increased along with the demand for its services. Supplies are endless and are an important part of the trade. The manicure alone is no longer enough to satisfy the needs of public demand. Nail extensions are increasing in popularity as are the different supplies and procedures used to reinforce or add strength to nails. All of this makes the nail industry a multi-million dollar business.

Knowing everyone is different and has different needs makes determining the right nail service important. To do this, a knowledge and an understanding of each given nail service is important in succeeding in this business.

A full knowledge of manicure theory, sanitation, bacteriology, and proper procedure is crucial to promote healthy nails and cuticles.

Remember, product knowledge is a must in order to get the most beneficial use of the supplies you use and to avoid hurting the client and/or causing permanent damage.

Knowing all the services available will insure that you never have to turn a client away. Anyone should be able to come to you and say I have acrylic and I need a fill-in or, I need a maintenance manicure for my linen wrap.

A good nail technician can become a best friend to every client's hands. You are an artist creating a picture on a living canvas. Your art does not hang in one spot on a wall but is seen every place your client goes. Remember whether you do a manicure, sculptured nails, or decorate every nail with gold and gemstones, the value of your work is still the same, a work of art, a change for the better.

If you think of your work as art and do your best, the result will build your confidence as your ability grows. Compliments your clients receive about their nails can lead right to your profits. This proud feeling enables you to get better in a very rewarding business that you can turn into your own.

CHAPTER 1

Start
to
Succeed

INTRODUCTION

Many factors affect the success of a business, several of which you can directly control. For example, your attitude and personal appearance can affect owner/ client relations. Physical factors include the surroundings, the work area, and the record keeping. Learn how to use these factors to their best advantage.

Attitude

Your personal attitude should always be compatible to your clientele. Be charming and maintain a professional environment. This is important to get respect from clients and co-workers. Never put down another technician's work. Do not talk loudly about clients' nail problems; keep it personal and confidential.

If you do have a disagreement with a client remember it is better to give a little extra service, such as no charge for a tip, than to lose a client.

Personal Appearance

Appearance plays a big part in being accepted: You must be neat and well groomed to service people who are looking for that very thing. Wear nail polish and keep your nails in good shape. Wear hair out of the way and dress professionally. Bad breath from smoking or from strong foods can be offensive, so remember to be considerate.

Surroundings

When clients walk into a salon they need to feel comfortable and welcomed. Try to create a nice atmosphere that is relaxing and pampering for everyone. Play background music that fits the mood of the salon. Use plants and artwork for decorations and supply magazines and beverages for clients.

Setting Up the Work Area

The more organized you are, the easier is your job. Arrange your table so you know where everything is.

1. Keep supplies for each service in separate containers or drawers to avoid wasting time looking for something.
2. Find organizer boxes or trays that suit your needs.
3. Do not clutter your table. Put only what you need on the table top. Keep other supplies in the drawer until needed.
4. Nail polish can be stored in a display area instead of on your table.
5. A pad or pillow under the towel adds comfort to the client.
6. Paper towels or other disposable covers can protect your good towels from glue, acrylic, or polish.
7. Sanitation supplies must be on your table at all times and used before each client. This is the law. You should also sanitize your table by wiping the table clean with an antiseptic spray. The clients' chairs also need to be maintained.
8. Have extra supplies on hand so you always have what you need for every service offered.

Appointment Book

When booking appointments always write clearly. Other people may have to read it. Always print both first and last names of every client and phone numbers, allowing you to call the client for any reason. Some reasons to call might be: if you are running late you can call the following appointment and ask her or him to come a little later, a missed appointment can be called to reschedule, or someone can be called to fill a canceled appointment. To schedule a new client get the address to add to a client service card later.

Be sure to write the correct service for each appointment. Some take longer than others and need to be scheduled accordingly. It can be upsetting if a client expects a manicure and four tips and you only can do a manicure. To please that client you will likely be late for the next one.

Make sure time is left between every client to sanitize table and implements.

Mark each client's appointment with the number of arrival after they arrive. This shows they made the appointment and at the end of the day the last appointment has the number of clients you did that day.

It is best to confirm all appointments. The morning appointments should be called on the evening before. The afternoon and evenings appointments should be confirmed the morning of the same day. This system is an efficient way to remind any forgetful clients. Put a "C" next to the confirmed appointments to indicate confirmation.

Book your appointments close enough together that you don't have big gaps between appointments. Get as much work in as possible without overbooking yourself. Be sure to leave time for lunch and time to clean your station appointments.

The person who books your appointments must know how long it takes for each service. For your own good, make sure the receptionist knows, or do it yourself if possible. Some salons don't allow anyone behind the front desk, except the receptionist. If they cannot book you correctly, then take the problem to your boss (who hopefully is not the receptionist).

Your appointment book is the most important tool in making money. Don't let someone mess it up for you. Without clients it doesn't matter how good you are; you still won't make any money. The following list of abbreviations can be used in an appointment book.

Full Set of Nails   F.S.
Sculptured Nails   Sc.N.

Tips and Acrylic	T.A.
Linen and Tips	Lin. T.
Silk and Tips	Sk.T.
Silk Wrap on Natural Nail	S.W.
Linen Wrap on Natural Nail	L.W.
Fill-Ins	F.I.
Manicure	Man.
Hot Oil or Hot Cream Manicure	H.O. Man. or H.C. Man.
French Manicure	F. Man.
One Nail Tip	1N; 2N; 3N., and so on

Combine the abbreviations to come up with the appointment needed. For example, a full set of sculptured nails would be abbreviated F.S./Sc.N. A full set of silkwraps with nail tips would be F.S./Sk.T. One nail and a manicure would be 1N/Man.

CHAPTER 2

Supplies, Description, and Usage

INTRODUCTION

The following list itemizes and describes the supplies necessary to adequately provide advanced nail techniques.

Supplies for Manicures and Advanced Nail Techniques

Acetone—This is used as the base ingredient for most nail polish removers. It is also used for dissolving nail glue, tips, acrylic, and other bonding materials. This product is flammable and should be stored in a cool place with a tight lid because it evaporates easily.

Acrylic—Most acrylic nail products available on the market consist of *polymers* (powders) and *monymers* (liquids). When mixed together they harden in about one to three minutes.

The liquid (monymer) has a strong odor which can affect the technician. The vapors may cause burning, itching, and watering of the eyes; dizziness; headaches; nausea; burning of the nose, throat, and lungs; and swelling of nail beds and fingertips. Sometimes blisters will appear on the fingers or nail bed.

5

To lessen these problems a disposable face mask can be worn to avoid inhalation of the vapors and dust (caused from filing). Also an air filter should be installed for ventilation. To protect hands, plastic gloves or fingerguards can be worn.

Some customers may have an allergic reaction to the chemicals. Ask customers if they are sensitive to chemicals or have any allergic reactions. Signs of allergic reactions are irritations to the cuticle area, burning of the nail bed, or swelling of the finger. If these symptoms appear, the acrylic should be removed immediately.

The powder (polymer) is available in clear, pink, or white (Figure 2-1). The clear and pink can be used on the nail bed and over nail tips. The white is used to build the tip for sculptured nails.

FIGURE 2-1
Acrylic nail polymers.

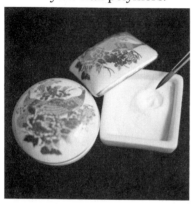

Alcohol—Used to sanitize all implements. Applied to the nail bed before the application of wrap, to clean the nail bed.

Antiseptic Soap—Used to clean hands and feet, antiseptic soap helps stop the spread of bacteria, infection, and germs.

Base Coat—A clear base coat is used under colored nail enamel. A good base coat can prevent stains on the nail bed from dark colors and helps the polish wear longer. A conditioning base coat can protect the nail from enamel drying it out.

Buffers—Buffers are used after shaping nails to smooth the surface. There are many types and shapes available: square, round, oblong, and rectangular. You always should try new kinds to find the one that gives you the best results.

Cotton Balls—Cotton balls are used saturated with polish remover or antiseptic.

Cuticle Massage Cream—Conditioning cream to massage into cuticles after a manicure or anytime to treat dry cuticles. Continued use helps maintain healthy nails and cuticles.

Cuticle Pusher—The cuticle pusher is used to push back the cuticle and carefully scrape the cuticle that is stuck to the nail bed. Scraping too hard can scratch the nail, causing a weak spot on the nail bed. Metal pushers are not recommended. Plastic or wood are less damaging to the natural nail.

Duster Brush—A contour brush or any stiff makeup brush can be used to remove dust from the nail bed after filing and before any product is applied. This is better than cotton because it leaves no cotton string on the nail bed. Use this tool after nails have been cleaned and *sanitized*. Wash with antiseptic soap daily.

Emery Block—Made of a sponge-like substance the emery block comes in several grades: soft medium, medium coarse, and medium fine. Gray in color, it can be used with oil and washed.

Feathers—Beautiful feathers are used like decals to decorate the nails. When combined with gems and stripes you can create beautiful designs.

Fiberglass Nail Wraps—A fiberglass mesh (Figure 2-2) is used to cover the nail bed and free edge of the nail. A special bonding resin that resembles thick glue is spread evenly over the fiberglass mesh, which is then sprayed with an activator that sets the resin and makes the glass mesh bond to the nail. The wrap is filed, then buffed.

Proper use of the fiberglass products is very important. A chemical reaction can cause a hot burning sensation to the client if used improperly. Also any nail bed that has been injured or recently broken, filed too thin, or is just plain sensitive can have a greater burn reaction. Every client must be aware of these possibilities. The heat sensation will subside almost as fast as it comes. Also tapping on the top of the nail bed with a orangewood stick will increase circulation and distract the discomfort. Test patches are recommended for anyone who is sensitive.

Files—There are many kinds of files, from very coarse to very fine (see Figure 2-3). The coarse file is best used on acrylic and for shaping nail tips, while the finer file is used to smooth the surface of silk or linen. Never use a worn out file; this can cause discomfort from friction.

Filler Powder—Fine powder in squeezable bottles is sprinkled onto glue to fill in space between the nail tip on the underside of the nail if needed, or to fill in the ridge between the nail and tip. Acrylic powder can be used in its place but both powders are hard to file.

Fingernail Brush—Small brush with a handle to scrub under the free edge and clean cuticles when manicuring or doing nail artistry.

Glue Setter—Glue setters enable the glue to dry instantly when wrapping or applying tips. They can be found in pump or aerosol sprays. The fast-drying action can make the nail bed burn if too much is used. Use caution—always spray very lightly. (To apply nail tips with setter, prepare nail plate, spray lightly, apply glue to nail tip, and press in place. It adheres instantly so be sure it is straight. Spray lightly after applying glue, then file.)

Gold Leaf—Gold leaf is available for applying to nails. You can get a beautiful gold nugget effect or a solid gold nail. It is applied with clear polish.

Light Nail Gel—This gel is applied to a nail tip to wrap a material nail or extend the nail using the sculptured nail method. This gel does not set until exposed to the light rays of a special ultraviolet lamp. Light nail gel is odorless; it should be used under specific instructions according to the system purchased. Heat sensation can occur on nail bed if used too thickly or if the nail is damaged.

Linen—Linen fabric (Figure 2-4) is applied with nail glue on natural nails for reinforcement. It is also used to wrap nail extensions. Linen is stronger than silk but does not look as natural. The linen is not

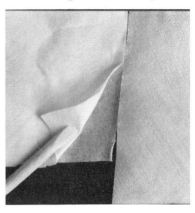
FIGURE 2-2
Fiberglass nail wrap.

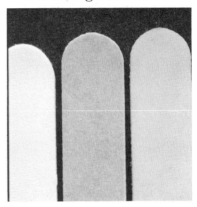
FIGURE 2-3
Different grades of files.

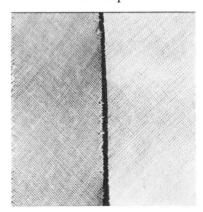
FIGURE 2-4
Linen fabric for nail repair or wrap.

transparent and cannot be worn without polish. When applied properly it should have a smooth finish. There are several types of linen being used. The linen fabric is actually cotton. The closer the weave the better. Pre-cut and strips or rolls are available.

Nail Clippers—Nail clippers come in two sizes, small and large. The small size is to cut fingernails and the large size is for the toenails. The toenail clippers are great for cutting nail tips when doing nail extensions.

Nail Gems—Nail gems come in many sizes, colors, and shapes. They are flat on one side and are easily set in clear polish to decorate nails.

Nail Glue—Nail glues are used for glueing on nail tips and applying linen or silk wraps. There are two types of glue: thin, fast-drying glue and thick, slow-drying. Glue will dissolve in regular polish remover or acetone.

Nail Polish Color—The color of polish used should enhance the appearance of the client's nails and skin tone. Most clients will choose their own color. Usually two coats are used. When completely dry, it can darken in color. Because nail polishes vary in price choose those that wear well on the *natural* nail.

Keep in mind that nails that are wrapped will hold the polish much longer because the polish is on a solid surface. When nail polish chips, it usually is because the nail itself has chipped or peeled, thus taking the polish with it.

Nail Tape—An adhesive tape in many colors and widths—the favorite color is gold in the thin strip.

Nail Tips—Nail tips are used to extend the free edge of the natural nail. Nail tips have numbers printed inside to indicate sizes. The sizes range from one through ten, one being the largest and ten the smallest.

Several types of nail shapes are available as well as types of plastics. Some nails are clear, yellow, hard, soft, thick, and thin. To best determine which to use try all that you can to see which is most comfortable for you.

The shape of the client's nail bed is an important determining factor in which type of nail tip to use. For this reason it is wise to have several types on hand to be sure you have a compatible shape for all clients.

No Light Gel—The gel used to coat the nail is thick and easy to control with an orangewood stick. After covering the prepared nail or nail extension an activator spray is used to set the gel and bond it to the nail. There are several systems on the market and more to come. Follow the procedures given for each system. Proper use can prevent any hot burning sensations to clients. Broken nails and sensitive nail beds can burn more. Clients should be told to expect it. The hot spot goes away almost as fast as it comes. If you tap on the top of the nail bed with an orangewood stick after spraying, circulation will increase and distract the heat sensation.

Always use great care when using any nail product that contains chemicals.

Non-acetone Polish Remover—This must be used on nails that are wrapped. It removes nail polish from fingernails without removing the wrap or tips. If regular remover or acetone is used the wrap or tip will either melt or lift away.

Orangewood Stick—The soft and splinterless orangewood stick is used to push back cuticles. It is also used when doing advanced nail techniques and nail art.

Pierced Nail Charm—A charm made smaller than usual with a screw-like stem on the back with a bolt. A special hand drill is used to make a small hole to hold the charm (Figure 2-5).

Primer—Nail primer is primarily made of acid. Its drying action removes the natural oils from the surface of the nail bed allowing the product to adhere to a dry, clean surface. This product must be used with careful attention. Too much primer can burn the nail bed and cause discomfort. Always avoid the skin and cuticle area; use very sparingly. The primer is applied only to the natural nail, not to the tip extension.

Quick Shine—This buffer can bring a quick shine to any nail surface by using the three different surfaces in order. One surface is slightly coarse, the second smooth (these two are half and half on one side). The remaining side is very smooth. When used in order—1, 2, and 3—the effect is great.

Ridge Filler—Ridge filler is used as a base coat. It is somewhat thicker than a regular base coat and has a light milky color. The thickness helps to fill in the ridges and scratches on the nail to make it smooth. This gives the polished nail a smoother look when done.

Sculptured Nail Forms—These are used to build acrylic extensions to the nail (Figures 2-6 and 2-7). The form is placed under the free

FIGURE 2-5
Pierced nail charm.

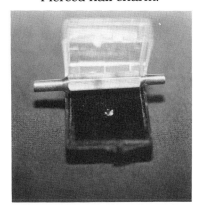

FIGURE 2-6
Sculptured nail forms.

FIGURE 2-7
Sculptured nail forms.

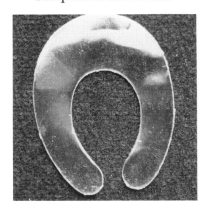

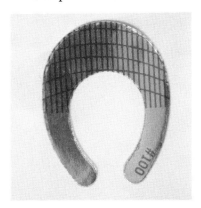

edge and attached to the finger at the sides. Then the acrylic is placed on the form to make the extension. Additional acrylic is placed over the nail bed and the extension to make the sculptured nail. A reusable form or a disposable nail form can be used. Try several types to find one that works best for you.

FIGURE 2-8
Silk fabric for nail repair or wrap.

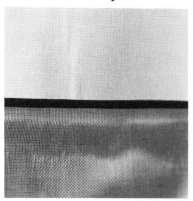

Silk—Silk fabric (Figure 2-8) is applied with nail glue onto the nail to reinforce the natural nail and nail extensions. Also silk can be used to repair split or peeling nails. Silk is not strong enough for ultra-long nail tips unless it is applied twice to add strength. Silk is available in pre-cut self-adhesive strips or in long strips or rolls.

Sterile Jar—Small jar used to store sterilization liquid. The jar should have a lid to prevent contamination when not in use. Some lids have an inside hook which can hang on the jar's edge to keep the lid close at hand. The lid should remain on the jar so it remains clean and nothing falls inside.

Top Coat—Top coat is used over colored enamel to protect it and maintain a high gloss appearance. It comes in clear or clear pink. The clear is used on most colors and the clear pink is mainly used on french manicures or just over a light pink or clear base coat for a natural look.

Ultraviolet Lamp—This lamp is used with light nail gel to set and bond the gel to the nail. The ultraviolet rays are safe. Any lamp used should be used only with products from that system.

Witch Hazel—Mild astringent that can be used to clean nail bed and refresh skin.

CAUTION: If too much glue is used the vapors can rise into your eyes and cause a temporary burning sensation. To avoid this do not hold your head directly over nails while applying glue to nails. Glue also can bond to skin quickly; be careful when using.

NOTE: Always use liquid at a warm temperature. When the room temperature is too cool the acrylic will not set properly and can crystallize. This product is flammable and should be kept away from heat.

Warnings on Chemical Products

Any product that is mixed with a chemical (even glue is a chemical) can cause a reaction of heat on the nail, a hot spot on the nail bed which burns, and can surprise or hurt clients especially if they are not aware that it is possible. To prevent such reactions follow all directions on all product packages. Misuse of any of these chemicals can be disastrous. Permanent damage can be caused to the nail bed along with the loss of a client.

To show clearly a sample of overusing a product carefully conduct this simple experiment:

Procedure

1. Take out the following supplies:

   Nail glue,
   Small plastic or glass container
   A quick dry/glue activator

2. Drop a large puddle of glue (six to ten drops) in the bottom of a dish.
3. Stand back, about arms length, from the dish and spray three or four pumps or for two seconds directly into glue.
4. Stand back and watch the reaction.

Glue should foam up when sprayed with activator. This foam is hot. Imagine it on a client's nail bed. After the foam cools and hardens pull it out with snippers to see the results.

Please read and follow all instructions on product packages. If you do not understand or if there is a problem call the manufacturer. They should offer a solution or try to help find an answer. If a company is not helpful try using another product. There are plenty to choose from.

CHAPTER 3

Preparing the Client for Services

Introduction

This chapter outlines the preliminary steps necessary for nail therapy. It also stresses the need to explain all services offered and to then personalize these services for each client.

Pre-Service Rules

Always exercise these pre-service rules before starting any type nail service on every client.

1. Follow all sterilization and sanitation rules. Wash your hands with antiseptic soap, have client wash hands with antiseptic soap, and sterilize all implements to be used.
2. Always sanitize each nail before applying any wrap and lightly roughen with soft file for clean surface.
3. Consult with clients about their individual needs and explain each service along with the benefits each has to offer. Help them decide which will be best for them (see client consultation section).
4. Check nails for any nail disorders and consult clients about necessary treatment if needed. If they have any contagious disorder do not service them. You can recommend they see a doctor and return after it has cleared up.

5. If doing any service that involves wrapping the nails or applying extensions you must ask your clients if they have any chemical allergies. Or, ask if they have sensitive skin. If they say yes, you should do a test patch to be sure they will not have a bad reaction from the products used on their nails. See the section on patch tests.

6. Before removing client's polish ask if they are wearing wraps or nail extensions. If they are, then do not use acetone base polish remover. Use polish remover for artificial nails only. This will avoid destroying the wrap or extension (see the section on removing nail polish).

7. If applying wraps or tips completely remove the old wrap in order for the new wrap or extension to adhere properly, unless you are doing a maintenance manicure or a fill-in.

8. Every client should be made aware of home-care rules to maintain perfect nails between visits. Be sure to give them do and don't rules along with nail care tips.

9. Explain basic mold or fungus possibilities if nail wraps and tips are not properly maintained. If new or current clients have mold ask them to cure it; they must follow close attention to keeping it bacteria free with antiseptic products.

Client Consultation

Before you can meet the need you must first find out what it is. When new clients sit at your table the first thing to do is consult with them about their needs. Some clients know exactly what they want and will tell you. Other clients may have no idea what they want or even what services are available. Explain each service and its purpose. Find out what length they desire and what shape they prefer. If a new client wants long nails and has never had them long explain that it is very different having long nails and can be very hard to adjust to. Suggest the client start with a moderate length and gradually increase nail length until the client is accustomed to having long nails. This will minimize breakage and make the transition to longer nails easier. Explain that this will help cut down on breaking nails that can lead to giving up on having long nails at all. Evaluate their nail conditions and suggest the technique most beneficial to their nail type and individual needs. Once you and your client have decided on the services needed—how long, what shape—explain what they need to know about caring for their nails once they leave. Chapter 13 covers home care.

To keep track of every client and all their special needs, a client consultation card can be made.

Every client should fill out the card on the first appointment during the consultation. The information will ensure quality service for them. You can record all the information about each individual so you do not forget any particular need. Getting the address and phone number on file is a great benefit of the card. Other information should include, nail evaluation, desired length, desired nail shape, size of nail tips used for each finger, wrap used, favorite nail polish color (see Figure 3-1).

Patch Test

Before you apply any wrap for the first time always test for sensitivity or allergic reaction. Using a nail wrap technique, do one nail and instruct client to carefully watch the nail for 24 hours. If nothing happens, then it is safe to complete the service. If any redness, swelling, or discomfort occurs any time after the patch was applied, it must be removed as soon as possible. Tell the client the proper way to remove the nail wrap without damaging the nail. Follow the instructions for removing wrap.

Points to Remember

1. Ask if the client is usually sensitive or has allergic reactions to anything. If extreme sensitivity does exist, you should stay with one chemical wrap that is easy to use such as silk or linen.
2. Never place the test patch close to skin. If irritation does occur it makes it harder to remove if it is near inflamed skin.
3. Be sure the client not only understands the importance of the test, but also how to remove it correctly at home if necessary.
4. List products needed at home to remove the test patch. If you do not sell the products suggest where they might be purchased.
5. If a client has any nail disorders that might worsen or if inflammation of surrounding tissue pus or swelling occurs you should refuse service at this time, recommend they see a doctor, and suggest they return after the condition is cleared up.

Client Consultation/Service Chart

Name _____

Phone _____

Address _____

Nail Shape _____ Desired Length _____

Nail Service _____

Nail Tip Size Chart

Right Hand: Thumb ____ First ____ Second ____ Ring ____ Pinky ____

Left Hand: Thumb ____ First ____ Second ____ Ring ____ Pinky ____

Evaluation / Comments _____

_____

_____

_____

FIGURE 3-1
Sample client consultation card.

Removing Nail Polish

The first step in nail treatment is cleansing the hands with antiseptic soap. Then the old nail polish can be removed and the nail surface cleaned. A cotton ball saturated with nail polish remover is rubbed over each nail to wipe away polish. Gauze pads can be used but cotton is more absorbent. When removing polish try not to spread it all over the finger. Be sure you remove all polish and residue stains that can be left from dark polish colors. If you are giving a manicure to a client with a wrap be sure to use a non-acetone polish remover. Acetone will loosen or destroy most wraps.

Procedure for Removing Polish

1. Gather the following supplies:

   Nail polish remover needed for service
   Cotton
   Orangewood stick/polish corrector
   Paper towels

2. Make a firm cotton ball about the size of a tablespoon.
3. Hold the ball between your first two fingers and thumb and squeeze the ball top while saturating the ball bottom with polish remover (Figure 3-2). If you are wearing nail polish you can hold the ball of cotton with the lower part of fingers and thumb instead of with your fingertips (Figure 3-3).

FIGURE 3-2
Proper way to hold cotton ball for polish removal.

FIGURE 3-3
How to hold a cotton ball when wearing nail polish.

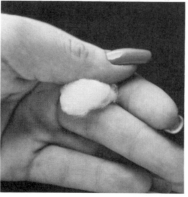
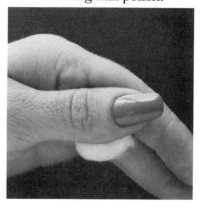

4. Squeeze any heavy drips off the ball bottom and continue to squeeze the ball top. Such squeezing keeps the polish remover at the bottom of the cotton ball where it is needed (Figure 3-4).

5. Place the ball on the lunula and move back and forth while moving down slowly to the end of the nail (Figure 3-5). A paper towel folded four times square can be placed under the hands to catch any drips.

FIGURE 3-4
Squeeze off excess polish remover drips.

FIGURE 3-5
Move bottom of cotton ball on lunula to remove polish.

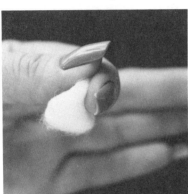
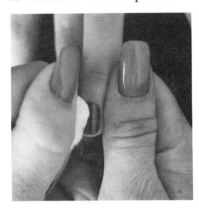

6. With thick polish, go over the nail several times to remove all the polish. When the cotton ball is full of polish and does not clean well, make a new ball. Sometimes a new ball must be made for each nail, while other times one ball for each hand will do.

7. Use nail polish corrector or an orangewood stick to clean nail grooves by dipping in polish remover. Twist the orangewood stick with a small amount of cotton at the end between fingers (Figure 3-6); then dip in polish remover and rub rest of polish off nails (Figure 3-7).

FIGURE 3-6
Cotton can be added to the orangewood stick.

FIGURE 3-7
After adding cotton, more remover is used to clean the nail.

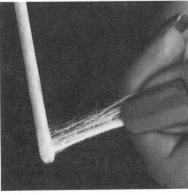
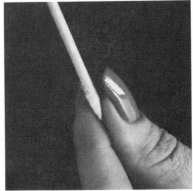

8. Proceed with manicure or desired nail service. If applying polish, next buff the nails lightly to stimulate circulation and to smooth nails.

Points to Remember

1. Follow pre-service rules.

2. Always ask clients if they are wearing wraps so you can use the correct polish remover.

3. Do not rub polish remover ball or pad all over the finger; stay on the nail to avoid staining the finger.

4. Be sure to check nail grooves and under free edges for traces of old polish.

5. Do not push too hard or dig polish stains from nail grooves or cuticles; a manicure should remove stains gently.

6. Hold remover pad correctly (not with your nails) to avoid ruining your own nail polish or wraps.

CHAPTER 4

Preparing the Nail for Advanced Techniques

INTRODUCTION

While file to use depends on what procedure the client is requesting. Choosing the correct file and learning how to hold the hand are discussed in this chapter. The techniques for filing and buffing are also explained step-by-step.

Filing Techniques

The main objective of filing nails is to create a natural shape. Every nail must be smooth and ridgeless. The length, width, and thickness are very important. Be consistent with your work. When you find something that works well for you stick with it; use the same technique on each nail.

The File

To get the best results from your file use a fresh one. A worn out file wastes time and creates friction and discomfort to the client. Always use the right file for the job: a coarse file for fast tip shaping, a medium file for shaping a wrap, and a soft file for a silk wrap or for smoothing the finish before buffing.

Holding the File

If right-handed, hold the file lengthwise between the first two fingers at right end. Let the thumb fall onto file near middle and bend just a little. Use the thumb to apply pressure to file. To use the arm would add much more pressure than needed. This can cause discomfort to the client or even damage the nail bed.

Bend your other two fingers into your palm to keep them out of the way, or hold them out straight to avoid hitting the client's fingers. If left-handed, apply the same method using the left hand.

To file the sides of a nail, hold the file's end between the thumb and bend the first finger (Figure 4-1). Bend the other fingers in to keep out of the way. Some people find it easier to use the thumb and first two fingers for a better grip on the file (Figure 4-2).

FIGURE 4-1
Proper way to hold a file.

FIGURE 4-2
An alternate way to grip a file.

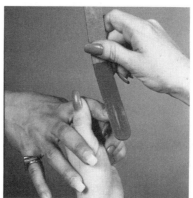
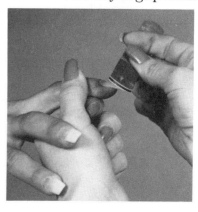

Holding the Client's Hand

Place thumb and first finger near the cuticle at sides of finger and gently pull the cuticle away from the nail to avoid hitting cuticle with file (Figure 4-3). Get a firm grip on client's finger but do not

FIGURE 4-3
Hold client's hand while filing.

FIGURE 4-4
Firmly grip the client's finger.

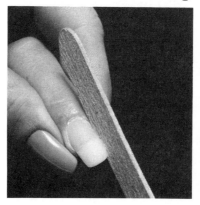
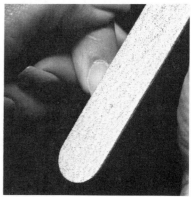

squeeze too hard. If filing the end of a long nail, you must support it at the breaking point and from underneath so it does not break (Figure 4-5).

Have the client put the fingers you are not working on out of the way so you don't hit them (Figure 4-6).

FIGURE 4-5
Support the nail at the underneath to prevent any breaks.

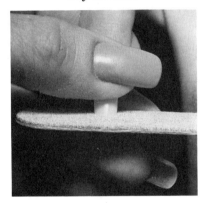

FIGURE 4-6
Keep the nail being filed clear of other nails.

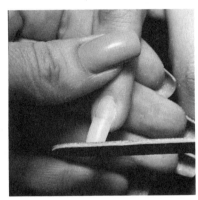

Filing

Before you begin filing check both sides of each nail tip to be sure that it is not glued to the side of client's finger (Figure 4-7). If it is, gently pry it away with an orangewood stick. If it does not separate easily, apply a small amount of acetone to the glued area using an orangewood stick or nail polish corrector pen. This will melt some of the glue, thus making it easier to separate.

Hold the file flat when filing on the tip or ridge (Figure 4-8).

FIGURE 4-7
Check both sides of each nail tip before filing.

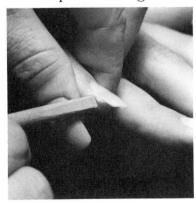

FIGURE 4-8
Filing on the tip or ridge.

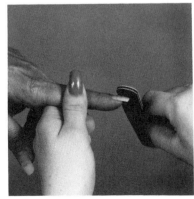

When filing the sides of nails, hold the file flat and straight, and line up the file with the nail groove for a guideline in shaping the sides (Figure 4-9). Use caution when filing near the nail groove (Figure 4-10). Put the pressure from the file on the side of nail, not into the nail groove to avoid cutting your client (Figure 4-11).

FIGURE 4-9
Filing on the sides of nails.

FIGURE 4-10
Be careful when filing near the nail groove.

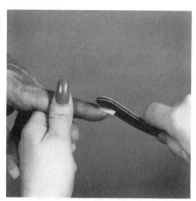

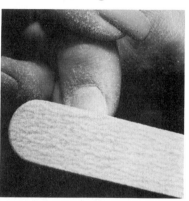

The filing movement is in the wrist not in the arm. Use the length of the file to make long, even strokes (Figure 4-12). To file with short jerky motions takes longer time and can cause pain to the client. Keep the file moving around the nail to avoid filing in one spot (Figure 4-13). Too much filing in one place can cause friction, resulting in a hot spot on the nail.

FIGURE 4-11
Pressure is placed on the side of the nail, not into the nail groove.

FIGURE 4-12
Use long even strokes when filing.

FIGURE 4-13
Move the file to avoid friction in any one spot.

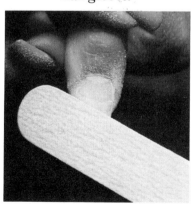

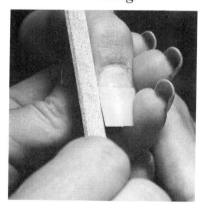

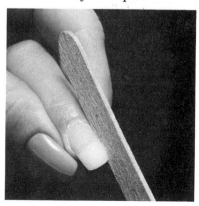

Never file on the natural nail with a heavy file. Keep the file on the nail tip or wrap only so you don't damage the natural nail.

After you achieve the desired shape, check each nail from the four angles of view to be sure the shape is correct and the same on each nail.

From the first angle, front view, look for the thickness of the nail and the evenness of the wrap at the free edge (Figure 4-14).

FIGURE 4-15
A second view is from the lunula to check the overall shape.

FIGURE 4-14
Front view of nail.

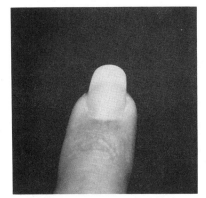

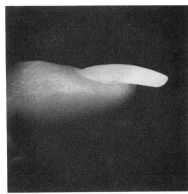

The second angle looks down the surface of the nail starting at the lunula to check the overall shape (Figure 4-15).

For the third angle, turn the finger sideways and look at the shape of the curve of the nail to be sure it is not bumpy and matches the other nails in shape (Figure 4-16).

Turn the finger to the other side for the fourth view and check it the same way as number three.

After you are sure the shape is correct buff the nails.

Buffing Techniques

FIGURE 4-16
Another view is to check the finger sideways.

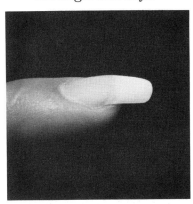

After the nails have been shaped with the file it is time to smooth the surface by removing the scratches made from the file. That is one reason why it is important not to use a very coarse file to finish shaping a wrap.

Always use a buffer that is not worn out or you will buff forever with no results. You do not save money buy using worn out buffers. Rather, you spend more time buffing instead of moving on to the next client and make more money in less time. In other words, you can actually lose money by not replacing worn out supplies.

Buffing

Hold the client's hand as you would for shaping the nail with a file. Use this technique with the buffer until all scratches are gone. If most of nail looks smooth and there is a big scratch or dip on the nail you can apply a coat of glue over the wrap to fill the spot. After it dries, buff it again.

Buff the under edges of nails as well as the top and check to see that the entire nail is smooth and free of snag spots (Figure 4-17). A nylon can be used to check for fingernail snags. Have clients check themselves by feeling fingernails with their fingertips.

Additional smoothing and shining can be achieved with finer grade buffers or quick shine buffers. Oil can be used in the final buff to help smooth the surface and at the same time to condition cuticles and to remove the dry look from fingertips (Figure 4-18).

FIGURE 4-17
Buff the edges and top
of the nail.

FIGURE 4-18
A smooth shine is achieved
with fine buffers or oil.

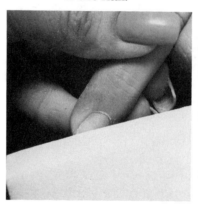

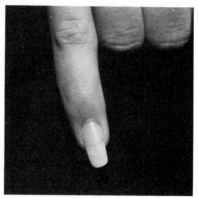

CHAPTER 5

Nail Tipping

INTRODUCTION

This chapter explains nail tipping which clients may want for various reasons, from extending nail length to cosmetic repair due to biting, chipping, or irregular nail shape.

Plain Nail Tipping

Nail tipping is done when one or all ten nails need to be lengthened. They can be temporary and easy to remove or made to stay by wrapping nails with silk, linen, acrylic, fiberglass, or gel bonding. For temporary tips no wrap is needed, and tips can be easily soaked off in acetone or tip remover.

Procedure for Nail Tipping

1. Take out the following supplies:

Nail glue	Orangewood stick
Nail tips	Large nail clippers
Rough file	Nail disinfectant
Buffer and swiss file	Duster brush

2. Trim natural nails so they are an even length and file the free edge to match the shape of the groove on the nail tip to be used (Figure 5-1).

3. Using an emery board, lightly roughen all ten natural nails. Dust with duster brush and disinfect the nail (Figure 5-2).

FIGURE 5-1
Trim the natural nails so they are even; then file them.

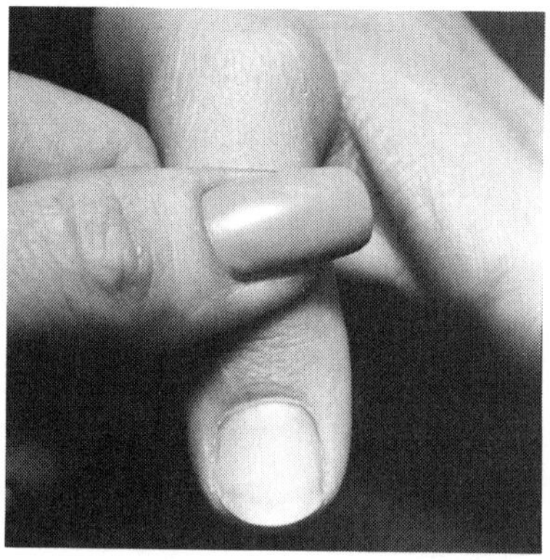

FIGURE 5-2
After filing, dust the nail with the duster brush.

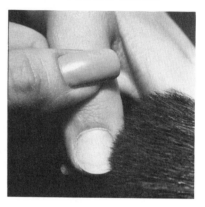

4. Select the tip sizes for all ten nails. The tips should be numbered to indicate sizes. When selecting size be sure the tip matches the width of the natural nail. It is better to cut down a tip that is too wide than to use one that is too small (Figure 5-3). However, make sure the tips are not too wide. This can cause discomfort to the client's nail by putting pressure on the cuticle or in the nail groove. (Refer to the section on cosmetic nail tips to work with crooked nail beds.)

5. Apply one drop of glue to base of the nail tip, holding the base down toward the table so the glue doesn't roll onto your fingers (Figure 5-4).

6. Place the base of the tip on the nail bed one-quarter of the way down and match the groove on the underside of the nail tip to the free edge (Figure 5-5), press the tip end down toward the table to make sure there is no space between nail's free edge and tip, and then press against the free edge. If nail glue doesn't dry, clean the nail and reapply using glue setter on natural nail.

FIGURE 5-3
Select a tip that matches the natural nail or cut a tip to fit.

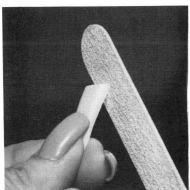

FIGURE 5-4
Glue is applied to the base of the nail tip. Be careful not to get glue on your finger.

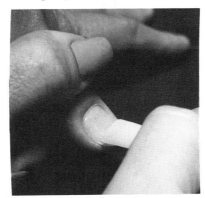

FIGURE 5-5
Place the nail tip on the nail bed and match the groove on the underside and press down.

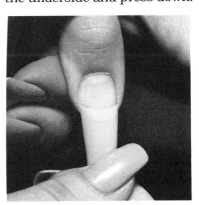

7. Use the nail clippers to cut the tips to desired length (Figure 5-6).

8. Shape the sides of each tip by holding the file straight. Use the line of the natural nail to determine width (Figure 5-7). The natural nail and the tip should be the same width (Figure 5-8). (See Chapter 4 for filing techniques.)

FIGURE 5-6
Use nail clippers to cut the tip to the desired length.

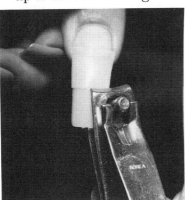

FIGURE 5-7
Shape the sides of each tip by holding the file straight.

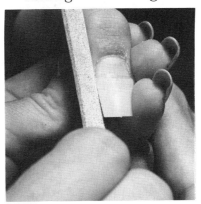

FIGURE 5-8
The natural nail and the tip should be the same width.

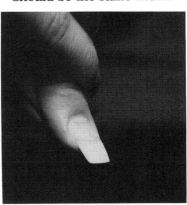

9. File the ridge of tip until smooth. Roughen the surface of tip, removing all shine (Figure 5-9).

10. Shape the end of the nail to achieve a round, oval, or square shape, whichever the client prefers (Figure 5-10).

FIGURE 5-9
File the tip ridge until smooth; then remove shine from the tip.

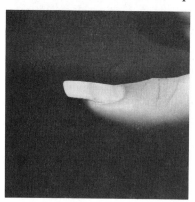

FIGURE 5-10
Shape the end of the nail to the desired shape.

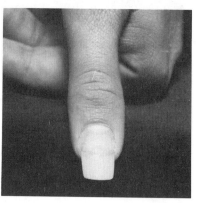

11. Brush off powder with duster brush.

12. For temporary tips, cover the entire tip and nail with three coats of glue, letting each coat dry in between.

13. If wrapping nails do so now (Figure 5-11).

14. File and buff smooth (Figure 5-12).

15. Manicure and polish.

FIGURE 5-11
Tips can be wrapped after dusting.

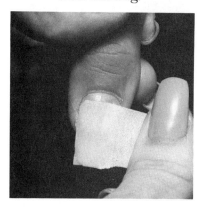

FIGURE 5-12
After buffing, nails can be wrapped.

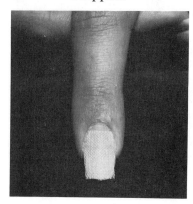

Points to Remember

1. Always suggest to clients who have never had long nails that long nails will be hard to get used to and will break easier.
2. When doing a full set of nails, cut natural nails to the same length so they can grow evenly.
3. Never glue the tip on too close to the cuticle or in the nail grooves.
4. Do not use too much glue.
5. Always tilt the nail tip down when applying glue.
6. Cut the nail tip as close to the desired length as possible to avoid excess filing at the nail tip.
7. Avoid any friction burn from too much filing.
8. Do not touch the nail bed with fingers to check ridge; use an orangewood stick.
9. Always check the nail to be sure it is perfect before wrapping with technique of choice.

Nail Tipping for Nail Biters

This service to most people is truly amazing. Nail biters usually have had the habit for many years or all their lives. Most don't remember what it is like to have fingernails of any length. Keep this in mind when determining the length. For the first time client, it is best to keep the nails as short as possible (Figure 5-13). Nail biters should always start with a short length and grow into a longer length to gradually adjust to the increased length. Explain that longer nails break more easily than short nails and if they are not used to ever having long nails they could have more breaks than usual. Such breakage becomes discouraging and may lead to giving up on trying to have nice nails. Be sure to give nail care tips.

Procedure for Nail Tipping for Bitten Nails

1. Take out the following supplies:

Nail glue	Orangewood stick
Nail tips with oval base	Large nail clippers
File	Duster brush
Buffer	Disinfectant

2. With an orangewood stick gently push back cuticles as much as possible. Do not push too hard.

FIGURE 5-13
Nail biters and first-time clients should start with a short nail length.

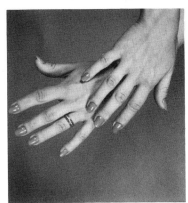

3. Use a file to roughen the nail bed (do not file on moon). Pay close attention to the sides and end of nails.

4. Dust nails with duster brush and disinfect nails.

5. Select the tip size for all ten nails. Make sure the tip covers the natural nail's width. With nail biters it is even more important that the tip fits perfectly. Remember, it is better to adjust an oversize tip than to use a tip that is too small. Check tip width; too wide tips can cause pressure on the cuticle or in the nail groove.

6. Now adjust the base of the nail tip to fit the length of client's nail bed (Figure 5-14). Hold the nail tip over the nail it is to be glued on. Match the groove on the underside of the tip to the edge of the client's nail. If nail is bitten too short then place the nail tip as closely as possible to where it should be. In some cases, part of the end of finger will be glued to tip along with the nail. This cannot be avoided sometimes but it will grow out. Cut the excess nail base off with clippers (Figure 5-15). This would be any part of tip that covers the moon on the client's nail bed. If the tip corners touch the cuticle at the nail base it can be trimmed slightly for a perfect fit. Do this to each nail tip.

FIGURE 5-14
Adjust the base of the nail tip
to fit the nail bed.

FIGURE 5-15
Cut off any excess nail base.

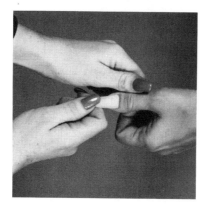
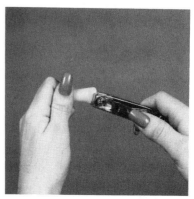

7. Apply one drop of glue to the base of the nail tip holding the base down toward the table so the glue doesn't roll onto your fingertips. Place the base of the tip on the nail bed and match the groove on the tip's underside to the free edge. Press the tip end down toward the table to make sure the edge is filled with glue. Lift the end of tip up slowly while watching the glue under the tip to be sure you don't force all the glue out from under the nail tip. It is fine and sometimes unavoidable to glue the nail onto the exposed skin on top of the finger where natural nail growth would normally cover.

8. Use the large nail clippers to cut nails to desired length.

9. Carefully file the free edge to the desired shape. Try to avoid filing on the skin at finger's end. Hold the file flat across the nail below the ridge and file the ridge as smoothly as possible without filing on client's skin. Nail biters usually have cuticle disorders from their biting. You certainly don't want to make it worse.

10. Cover the nail with glue. Use the orangewood stick to apply glue to area near cuticle. Let dry. Do this three times to build a layer of glue on the surface of nails.

11. File the surface again to ensure a smooth and natural shape.

12. Buff nails now. For more strength on long nails a wrap can be applied. For men, the silk is used because of its transparency. For women, linen or silk can be used if they wish to wear nail polish (Figure 5-16).

FIGURE 5-16
After wrapping, the nails can be polished.

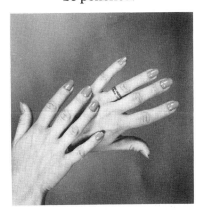

> **NOTE:** Acrylic is not recommended on nail biters unless they plan to continue the wrapping service to grow longer nails.

Points to Remember

1. Do not make their nails long.
2. Fingertip length is best until the natural nail has a chance to grow longer for more support.
3. Always give strict instructions not to bite or pick at tips and cuticles or any part of fingertips.
4. Maintenance manicure is required every week until the natural nail reaches the end of the fingertip.

Cosmetic Nail Tipping

When a client has a deformed nail it can sometimes be corrected by applying a tip in such a way to appear normal. A crooked nail can be made straight or a severe concave nail surface can be made to look flat, even curved if desired.

Procedures to Straighten Nails

1. Take out all supplies needed for nail tipping and wrapping.
2. Follow instructions for nail tipping up to step 3.
3. Before gluing on nails, look at the finger and hand. Determine the direction the nail would go if it was growing straight (Figure 5-17). This is the angle you use to glue the tip on. It will be crooked according to the direction of the natural growth. It will look straight when looking at the hand (Figure 5-18).
4. Now follow the remaining nail tipping procedures, starting at step 4 (Figure 5-19).

FIGURE 5-17
Carefully determine the direction of nail growth in a crooked nail.

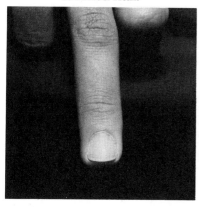

FIGURE 5-18
The nail should appear straight when looking at it.

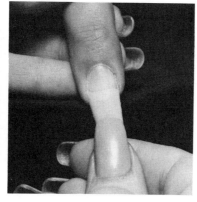

FIGURE 5-19
Once the tip is glued and filed, wrapping can begin.

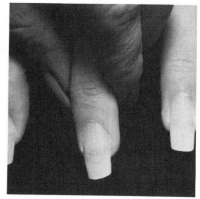

Points to Remember

1. Never apply a tip to a badly damaged nail that looks tender or has not healed.
2. Always inform client that the nail grows crooked and this is temporary until it grows out and then it must be done again. Because no two crooked nails are the same always treat each nail individually.

Procedures for Filling in Concave Nails

1. Take out all supplies needed for nail tipping and wrapping and filler powder.
2. Follow instructions for nail tipping up to step 3.
3. Select the tip to be used and cut a "V" shape in the base of the nail. This will allow the sides of the tip to be glued properly to the sides of the nail, while leaving the center open and free of air bubbles. This area will be filled in later.
4. Continue nail tipping instructions from step 4 through step 9. Be careful not to overfile. There will be a ridge and a dip in the nail center where filing powder will accumulate. Don't brush the powder; leave it in the center dip and add glue to fill area. If the area is not filled enough, add filler powder to fill in completely. Then apply more glue. Be sure all the powder is absorbed with glue. This can be done three or four times if the dip is real deep. Do not use too much filler powder and glue at one time. A little bit at a time is better. Also do not overfill area or you will have to file too much. Let dry.
5. File nail surface to achieve a smooth natural shape.
6. Dust nails and apply wrap of choice.

Points to Remember

1. Do not use too much filler in dipped area to avoid overfiling.
2. It is better to go back and add filler than to have too much at one time.
3. Avoid using too much glue.
4. Always clean excess filler from the nail groove and cuticle before gluing.
5. Be gentle with concave nails as they are usually sensitive.
6. When choosing a wrap keep in mind client's individual needs such as length and strength of nails.
7. Do not overfile nails.

CHAPTER 6

Nail Wraps

INTRODUCTION

Nails can be wrapped in a variety of ways. The strong linen wrap and the more fragile but more natural looking silk wrap are the most popular techniques. Fabric wraps can be used to strengthen and straighten long natural nails. This and the techniques of fiberglass wrapping are explained. Maintenance manicures are necessary to keep the nails strong and lasting.

Linen and Silk Fabric Wraps

Wrapping nails with linen and silk fabric reinforces and protects the natural nail or nail tip extension. Linen is stronger than silk, is whitish in color, and is hard to see through to check nail condition. Holding unpainted nails up to a lamp will light the fingers sufficiently to see if there is any discoloration that might indicate a fungus or mold. The thickness of linen makes it stronger than silk. It is great for long nails and for wrapping nail tips. If the natural look is not for you and you want a strong fabric wrap then linen is the best.

Silk is less durable because it is thinner. It becomes almost clear when glued to the nail. It is perfect for short or medium length nails and for clients who prefer a natural look. If long nails are done in silk because the client likes french manicures or wears clear polish for a natural look, you can layer the silk three or four times to make it stronger. If a natural look is not important, then it is better to use linen. One or two layers of linen is stronger and less time consuming than several layers of silk.

34

When filing on linen, remember it is thicker and a little harder than silk and needs more filing. The silk is thin and requires little filing with a lighter touch.

Be sure all of fabric linen or silk is completely absorbed with glue and check for air bubbles. Anytime you see a light or whitish spot it indicates a need for more glue. Always apply glue sparingly to avoid getting on skin. All fabric must be pressed smooth and flat to the nail and not on the cuticle or nail groove or it will cause lifting of wrap. Wrap left in the nail groove can cause pressure and discomfort to clients. Always do a neat clean job.

Procedure for Fabric Wrap Technique 1

1. Take out the following supplies:

Manicure supplies	Plastic square
Thin fast-drying glue	(about 3 × 3 inches)
Linen or silk	Orangewood stick
Medium grade file and	Buffers
soft grade file	Duster brush
Small sharp scissor	Nail sanitation products

2. Follow pre-service rules.
3. Remove old polish and clean nails. Gently push the cuticles back.
4. Use fine file to shape free edge and lightly roughen the surface of nails. Do not file on nail surface. The purpose is to carefully take away the top dry layer of the nail which is very thin. This creates a new surface, not a rough scratched one. Pay close attention to the free edge and nail groove area. Do not touch the lunula or moon. Always practice the greatest care when it comes to the natural nail surface. This promotes healthy nails, not damaged ones.
5. Use a duster brush to clean powder from filing nails.
6. Sanitize nails with disinfectant and let dry.
7. If extending nails with nail tips, do so now (Figure 6-1).
8. Prepare fabric for application by cutting the upper corner of strip making it round to match the shape of the nail bed and cuticle (Figure 6-2). The side that goes next to nail groove should be trimmed straight.
9. Hold the finger firm at a downward angle with the free edge pointing to the table. This keeps any excess glue from running into the cuticle when applying it. Gently pull the cuticle back at sides and hold.
10. Apply one drop of glue to the center of free edge.

FIGURE 6-1
Prepare to apply the silk wrap.

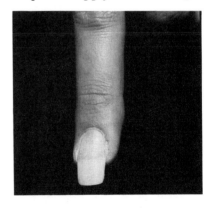

FIGURE 6-2
The fabric should match the shape of the nail bed.

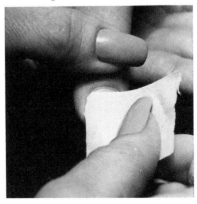

11. Set fabric on nail just below the lunula. Line the fabric up with the nail groove making sure the pre-cut side is completely covering nail but, not overhanging on skin (Figure 6-3).

12. Use plastic between wrap and your finger to press and rub the fabric flat and smooth on nail (Figure 6-4). Press the sides and end of free edge to secure fabric. The plastic should not stick to glue. If it does, you can file it off. If you have a problem with glue sticking to your plastic, try a thicker type. Always use clear plastic so you can see what you are doing.

FIGURE 6-3
Line the material up with the nail groove.

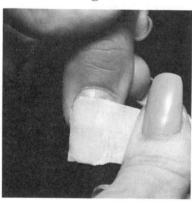

FIGURE 6-4
Use plastic to press fabric flat onto the nail.

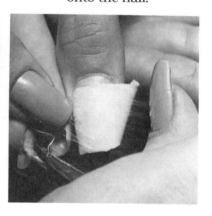

FIGURE 6-5
Apply glue to entire wrap to completely saturate the wrap.

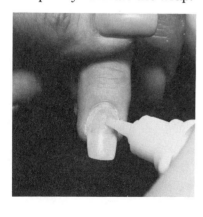

13. Remove plastic and carefully trim excess fabric. Do not trim sides too short. Hold the bottom of scissor on nail groove for a guideline or press top of fabric with an orangewood stick in the nail groove lightly to make a mark on fabric for a guide. Trim evenly and do not leave any overhang on skin. Trim the corner to match shape of cuticle.

14. Apply more glue to the entire wrap to completely saturate fabric (Figure 6-5). Do not put too much glue or it will run onto cuticles or under nail. Use an orangewood stick to press sides in place while drying. Plastic can be used again if majority of wrap needs to be pressed down.

15. Quickly remove any excess glue from cuticle and underneath nail. Let dry. If you need to speed up the drying time an instant glue setter can be used; hold it six inches or more from nail and sparingly spray a fine mist. (Read instructions on container.)

16. Use a medium file to smooth the ridge at the nail base, avoiding filing on the lunula (Figure 6-6). Hold the file straight and shape the sides of wrap; then lightly file surface until bumps are gone (Figure 6-7).

FIGURE 6-6
Use a medium file to smooth out the base of nail.

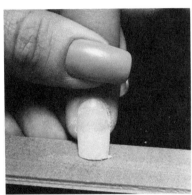

FIGURE 6-7
All bumps on nail should be filed away.

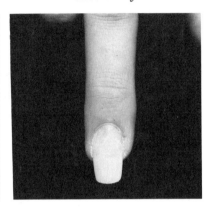

17. Apply another coat of glue and spread it evenly with the orangewood stick (Figure 6-8). Check both sides and the free edge to be sure all is secure. Let dry.
18. Use fine file to smooth the wrap, shape free edge, and bevel end of nail.
19. Buff nail until completely smooth (Figure 6-9).
20. Continue onto next service, manicure, polish, or nail art (Figure 6-10).

FIGURE 6-8
Apply another coat of glue and spread with an orangewood stick.

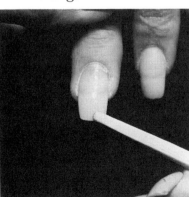

FIGURE 6-9
Buff the nails until smooth before starting manicure.

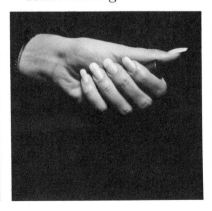

FIGURE 6-10
Continue with manicure, polish, or nail art.

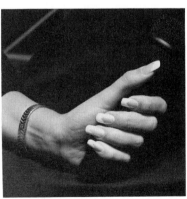

Points to Remember

1. Don't cover the lunula.
2. Do not use too much glue; let glue get in nail groove or cuticle. If glue hardens in nail groove it can sometimes be clipped out carefully. Also acetone or glue remover can be dropped on the area to loosen the glue first; then scrape or clip gently.
3. Do not harm the nail groove by digging.
4. Never file on the nail bed.
5. When roughening nail bed, use light pressure and exercise great care in avoiding lunula and cuticle.
6. Trim edges before applying more glue.
7. If using silk, one layer at a time can be applied if folding technique is difficult; two or more layers of silk are needed for a strong wrap. Linen needs one layer for short or medium lengths, and two or more layers for longer nails needing more support.
8. Do not overfile silk or it will weaken from being too thin. Linen requires more filing to ensure smoothness, while too much filing in one spot for too long will cause friction and burn client's nail bed.
9. Check for bumps with your fingers; sometimes you can feel bumps easier than you can see them.
10. Always check cuticles and under nails to be sure the area is clean.

Alternate Wrap Technique

If you don't like to use the plastic method you can apply the fabric wrap this way just as quick when you get the knack, by pulling the fabric gently while setting it in the glue you cause a sponge like effect and more glue gets absorbed into the fabric.

Both wrapping techniques are easy and quick to do. Try both of them to see what works better for you.

Procedure for Fabric Wrap Technique 2

1. Take out the following supplies (same as Technique 1):

Manicure supplies

Thin fast-drying glue

Linen or silk

Medium grade file and
soft grade file

Small sharp scissor

Plastic square
(about 3 × 3 inches)

Orangewood stick

Buffers

Duster brush

Nail sanitation products

2. Follow steps 1 to 6 for fabric wrapping techniques.

3. Hold fabric of choice from both sides at the very edges of fabric. Hold the fabric with the side edge of the thumbs and the first finger bent in (see Figure 6-11).

4. Put a strip of glue down the middle of the nail, starting just below the lunula down to the free edge.

5. Set the fabric below the lunula while gently pulling it over the nail; pull down at the sides and gently pull it down over the free edge. Let dry for a minute.

6. Trim edges precisely by lining the scissors up with the nail groove. Don't let any fabric hang over onto nail and do not cut it too short. The fabric must come to the edge perfectly.

7. Apply glue to nail and spread with an orangewood stick while pressing the edges down all around (Figure 6-12). If doing a large nail you can put glue on one side of the nail and press it into place. Then go to the other side and glue it. Let dry.

8. Continue following instructions for technique 1 from step 14 (Figure 6-13).

FIGURE 6-11
Hold the fabric with the side edge of the thumbs and the first finger bent in.

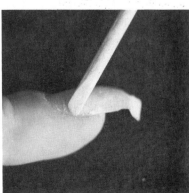

FIGURE 6-12
Use an orangewood stick to spread nail glue.

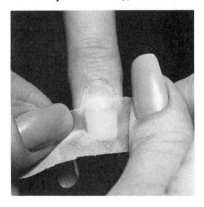

FIGURE 6-13
After glue dries, finish wrapping.

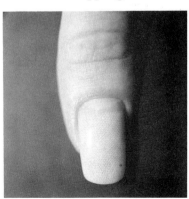

Points to Remember

1. Don't cover the lunula.
2. Do not use too much glue; let glue get in nail groove or cuticle. If glue hardens in nail groove, it can sometimes be clipped out carefully. Acetone or glue remover can be dropped on the area to loosen the glue first; then scrape or clip gently.
3. Do not harm the nail groove by digging.
4. Never file on the nail bed.
5. When roughening nail bed, use light pressure and exercise great care in avoiding lunula and cuticle.
6. Trim edges before applying more glue.
7. If using silk, one layer at a time can be applied if folding technique is difficult; two or more layers of silk are needed for a strong wrap. Linen needs one layer for short or medium lengths and two or more layers for longer nails needing more support.
8. Do not overfile silk or it will weaken from being too thin. Linen requires more filing to ensure smoothness, while too much filing in one spot for too long will cause friction and burn client's nail bed.
9. Check for bumps with your fingers; sometimes you can feel bumps easier than you can see them.
10. Always check cuticles and under nails to be sure the area is clean.

FIGURE 6-14
A wrap can be used to straighten a nail.

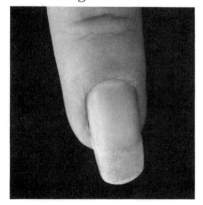

Straighten Long Natural Nails with Fabric Wraps

This process is done by wrapping the nail after adjusting it and pulling it straight. The wrap holds the new shape in place until it grows out. Your client must know it is only temporary. As the nail grows, it will take its natural shape and need to be redone. Fabric wraps are the best for this procedure. Linen is suggested because it is durable, strong, and easy to work with. To straighten a nail that is already wrapped you must first remove the wrap completely and start fresh (Figure 6-14).

Procedure to Straighten Long Natural Nails

1. Take out the following supplies:

   Linen wrap supplies
   Non-stick plastic

2. Follow pre-service rules.

3. Remove old nail polish and clean the nails. Gently push cuticles back with the cuticle pusher.

4. Check nails for any breaks, cracks, and lifting around the edges, especially the sides of free edge at breaking point. This area is usually the first to get damaged because it receives the most wear and tear. If there are any repairs to be done it should be done now. (See the section on nail patching and repairs.)

5. File wrap lightly with medium file to remove residue from polish remover. Sometimes stain is left from a dark colored polish. A new clean surface is what you want before glue can be applied. Do not file on the new nail growth and lunula. Gently buff to clean surface.

6. If the nail is slightly irregular and pliable, you can first try gently pulling on the free edge to straighten the nail. If this does not work, then make a tiny angular nip inside of nail where the curve or twist is. Additional nips can be made where needed to let the nail give when pulling straight. *Never* make nips straight across from each other, too close, or horizontally; this will weaken the nail too much.

7. Cut the linen end to fit the nail bed perfectly on both sides like a tab or tongue. You can mark your cutting lines by placing the linen just below the lunula and gently rub an orangewood stick in the nail groove on the linen making a wrinkle mark to follow for a perfect fit when you cut.

8. Apply a drop of glue to a pre-cut end of linen and set it on the nail bed just below the lunula. This attaches the wrap securely so you can pull the nail straight.

9. Apply a thin strip of glue down the nail middle and pull on the end of the linen. Use an orangewood stick to support the nail out straight. Hold until set.

10. Trim all edges of linen precisely to the edges of nail.

11. Put plastic on table under the nail, turn palm of hand up, and apply glue to one side of nail. Be sure to get glue between linen and nail. Turn nail to side and set on plastic while pressing nipped area flat with an orangewood stick. After it is smooth and dry the other side can be done in the same way. When done, pull the plastic off (Figure 6-15). If plastic sticks it can be filed off easily.

FIGURE 6-15
Gently and firmly pull plastic from nail.

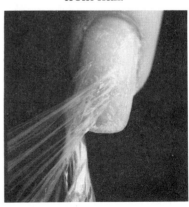

12. Turn palm down and apply glue to top of nail and smooth down with an orangewood stick.

13. Let dry or lightly spray with a glue setter.

14. Shape wrap with medium file. Do not overfile the edges.

15. Be sure bumps are gone and ridge is smooth; then apply more glue to top of wrap and under edges.

16. While drying, check under edge nip areas with an orangewood stick to be sure they are secure. If needed, a tiny amount of filler powder can be sprinkled on uneven surface of underside of nail.

17. Buff top of nail and under edge until smooth. Try folding the buffer to get under the nail better.

Points to Remember

1. Do not make nips too big.

2. Always nip at a angle, never straight across a nail.

3. Pull gently on nail to avoid breaking it.

4. For extra long nails additional layers of linen can be added for greater strength.

5. The more layers, the thicker it will be.

6. Do not use too much filler powder under the nail.

7. Clean any excess glue before it dries.

8. Support the nail with orangewood stick while pulling it straight.

9. If you need to hold the nail while straightening, use plastic on your fingers to avoid sticking.

Fiberglass Nail Techniques

Fiberglass nail wraps, one of the newest methods of nail services, are remarkably stronger and lighter than other nail enhancing products.

The fiberglass is actually a mesh made of fine fiberglass. Combined with a bonding resin and a special activator the mesh turns into a clear, strong coating over the nail or nail tips.

This method can be used on almost any client to strengthen natural nails or apply over nail tips. Because of the chemical change that takes place on the nail, discomfort can occur to sensitive fingers. Always recommend a test patch to new fiberglass clients. Show them how to remove it properly if they have a bad reaction.

Procedure for Fiberglass Wrap on a Natural Nail

1. Take out the following supplies:

   Manicure supplies   Activator
   Self-adhesive fiberglass mesh Files
   Bonding resin   Buffer

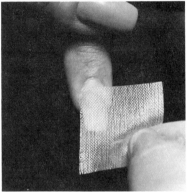

FIGURE 6-16
Cut the mesh to fit over the nail.

2. Remove old polish. Wash hands with antiseptic soap and water only. Do not use anything on nails after washing—no acetone, alcohols, or other nail cleaners.
3. Dry each nail completely with a clean cloth or pad. Cotton and tissue can leave residue.
4. Cut mesh to fit over nails to be covered (Figure 6-16). Leave 1/16 of an inch from all edges.
5. Avoiding the cuticle, press self-adhesive mesh firmly and smoothly over each nail (Figure 6-17). Be sure there are no bumps or bubbles under mesh. Trim any hang over of mesh from the free edge, cuticle, and nail groove.

FIGURE 6-17
Press self-adhesive mesh firmly and smoothly over the nail.

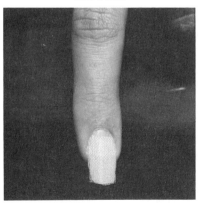

FIGURE 6-18
Add bonding resin to fiberglass mesh.

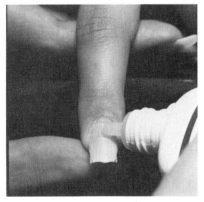

FIGURE 6-19
Spread resin with an orangewood stick.

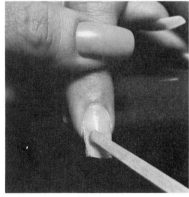

6. Apply a thin coat of bonding resin evenly over fiberglass mesh and spread with an orangewood stick (Figures 6-18 and 6-19). Always avoid the cuticle. Any product left on the cuticle or skin must be removed completely before the next step. If left, it will be hard to remove and even cause discomfort to the client.
7. Hold the activator spray at least 12 inches over nail and spray lightly. Too much spray can cause a heat reaction.

8. Apply a second coat of bonding resin thinly and evenly over nail (Figure 6-20). Remove from cuticle and nail grooves.
9. Spray again with activator from at least 12 inches away from nail.
10. File nail to desired shape and length. Smooth the sides and blend the product line at the nail base (Figure 6-21).

FIGURE 6-20
Bonding resin should be applied thinly and evenly over nail.

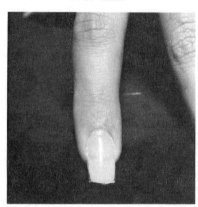

FIGURE 6-21
File nail to desired length and shape.

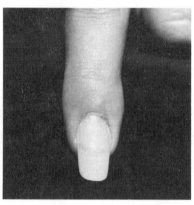

11. If dips on the surface occur, a third application of bonding resin and activator spray can be applied.
12. Buff nails to a glossy finish.
13. Clean cuticles and hands before start of polishing or nail art service.

Points to Remember

1. Do not get fiber mesh on cuticles or in nail grooves; put it $\frac{1}{16}$ of an inch from edges.
2. Never cover the lunula.
3. If activator spray is held too close to nail a chemical reaction can make the nail bed burn.
4. Do not touch skin with bonding resin or spray.
5. Use non-acetone polish remover to remove polish.

Procedure for Fiberglass Wraps Over Tips

1. Take out the following supplies:

Manicure supplies   Activator spray
Nail tips   Files
Fiberglass mesh   Buffer
Bonding resin

2. Remove old polish. Wash hands with soap and water only. Do not use anything on nails after washing—no acetone, alcohols, or other nail cleaners.

3. Dry each nail completely with a clean cloth or pad. Cotton and tissue can leave residue.

4. To assure the stability to the natural nail apply a thin, even coat of bonding resin to the natural nail. Allow the $\frac{1}{16}$-inch space around the nail edge.

5. Spray with activator, holding it at least 12 inches from nail to avoid burning. This will support the nail and tip by creating a stronger base for holding the nail tip.

6. Lightly file the surface to a dull finish. A lightweight file gives best results.

7. Select nail tips and sizes. Get them ready to apply after next step.

8. Apply bonding resin to the end of nail where tip is to be attached.

9. Apply tip to nail by pressing it into the bonding resin. Too much pressure will cause air bubbles. If this happens, remove the tip, clean the nail, and reapply. Any bonding resin that escapes must be removed from skin.

10. After 10 to 15 seconds spray lightly with activator at least 12 inches away.

11. Apply a small amount of bonding resin to seam, avoiding the cuticle, and blend seam with an orangewood stick.

12. Spray activator lightly from 12-inch distance.

13. Cut tip to desired length.

14. With a medium grade file, shape nail tip and blend seam into the natural nail. Be sure there is no ridge left or bump from nail tip before the next step. The surface shape now determines how smooth the finished work will be.

15. Cut self-adhesive mesh to fit the nail. Leave $\frac{1}{16}$ of an inch area border around cuticle.

16. Press mesh into place. Be sure there are no bubbles or bumps.

17. Apply a thin coat of bonding resin evenly over the glass mesh. Use an orangewood stick to spread after applying. Always avoid the cuticle. Any product left on cuticle or skin must be removed completely before the next step. If left on, it will be hard to remove and will cause discomfort. If dips in

the surface of nail occur, a second application of bonding resin and activator spray can be applied.

18. Finish with steps 10 and 11 of fiberglass on natural nails.

19. Hold the activator spray at least 12 inches over nail and spray lightly. Too much or too close can cause a heat reaction.

20. Apply a second coat of bonding resin thinly and evenly over nail. Remove any from cuticle and nail grooves.

21. Spray again with activator from 12 inches away.

22. File nails to desired shape and length.

23. Smooth the sides and blend the line at the nail base.

24. If dips on the surface occur, a third application of bonding resin and activator spray can be applied.

25. Buff nails to a glossy finish.

26. Clean cuticles and hands before start of polishing or giving nail art.

Points to Remember

1. Do not get fiber mesh on cuticles or in nail grooves; put in $\frac{1}{16}$ of an inch from edges.

2. Never cover the lunula.

3. If activator spray is held too close to nail a chemical reaction can make the nail bed burn.

4. Do not touch skin anywhere with bonding resin or spray.

5. Use non-acetone polish remover to remove polish.

Maintenance Manicure for Nail Wraps

After a wrap has been on the nails for a week or so the sign of growth is showing. A manicure is recommended once a week. Along with a manicure you maintain the wrap by checking it for lifting or cracks and then reglue the wrap after any repairs are done. If the nails have week-old polish, you can see clearly how much the nail has grown. Because the wrap is attached to the nail it moves forward as the nail grows. Securing the wrap with glue maintains the nail or wrap, thus making longer lasting and stronger nails. All signs of loose wrap are easy to see because lifting area turns white. When properly glued it will darken as the glue runs back under the edges and secures it.

Procedure for Maintenance Manicure

1. Take out the following supplies:

   Manicure supplies   Orangewood stick
   Thin fast drying glue   Buffers
   Medium grade file and   Duster brush
       soft grade file   Nail sanitation product
   Small sharp scissor

2. Follow pre-service rules.
3. Remove old nail polish and clean nails. Gently push cuticles back with the cuticle pusher.
4. Check nails for any breaks, cracks, or lifting around the edges, especially the free edge sides at breaking point. This area is usually the first to get damaged because it receives the most wear and tear. If any repairs are needed do it now. (See the section on nail patching and repairs.)
5. Buff the wrap with a medium file to remove residue from polish remover (Figure 6-22). Sometimes stain is left from dark colored polish. The surface must be clean before glue can be applied. Do *not* file on the new nail growth and lunula.
6. Use a duster brush to clean powder from filing off nails.
7. Sanitize nails with disinfectant and let dry.
8. Hold the finger and firmly pull the cuticle back at sides. While holding the cuticle back, point the nail down to the table to keep any excess glue from running into the cuticle when applying it. Start at the top of nail and let glue run under the wrap edges where color is light or whitish. You can see the glue fill the needed area. Then apply glue to entire surface of wrap. Avoid the lunula and cuticles. Get close to the edges without touching them by using the orangewood stick to spread.
9. Turn palm up to check the underside of nails. Apply glue with an orangewood stick to the free edge. To do this apply one drop of glue to the stick end and touch the wrap where it meets the natural nail or tip. Apply glue in this manner to all edges of wrap to ensure it is sealed. If you use the tip of the glue bottle to spread glue it can come pouring out and create a mess. It is better to be safe and in control than to waste valuable time cleaning an avoidable mess.
10. Apply a second coat of glue, using same technique. Let dry.
11. Buff nails until completely smooth (Figure 6-23). Pay attention to edges.
12. Continue on to next service, manicure, polish, or nail art.

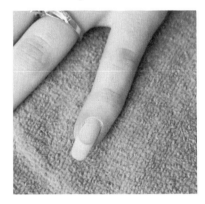

FIGURE 6-22
Buff the wrap to remove residual polish remover.

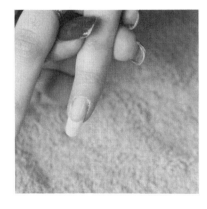

FIGURE 6-23
After the second coat of glue is dry, buff the nails until smooth.

Points to Remember

1. All polish and residue must be removed from nails before glue is applied.
2. All lifting wraps must be repaired properly.
3. It is better to remove a badly damaged wrap and replace it than to try and save it.
4. Glue should completely cover wrap.
5. Always glue the under *edge* of nails.
6. Do not glue the back of nail underneath.
7. Do not get glue on lunula, cuticle, or skin under nails.
8. Do not scrape or pry glue off the finger; use glue remover and gently rub it off.

CHAPTER 7

Acrylic and Sculptured Nail Techniques

INTRODUCTION

Acrylic is used to make sculptured nails, a process of building or extending the free edge with acrylic by placing a fitted nail form under the free edge to make a platform for the acrylic to set on. When dry, the form is removed and the new tip is left to be shaped by filing the edges and surface.

Another use for acrylic is to add strength to natural nails and nail tip extensions by covering them like a wrap. To maintain acrylic nails, fill-ins are needed when the nail grows and the natural nail is exposed half-way to the breaking point. (See Chapter 10 for fill-in techniques.)

Acrylic Over Natural Nails and Tip Extension

Covering the natural nails with acrylic and putting acrylic over nails with tip extensions is the same except for one thing: You lengthen nails by applying tip extension before applying the acrylic instead of putting the acrylic over the natural nail. The fill-in procedure is the same for both as well as sculptured nails.

The following acrylic techniques are for covering the natural nail and/or tips. If extensions are being used, refer to nail tipping techniques first.

Procedure for Applying Acrylic Over Natural Nail or Tip Extensions

1. Take out the following supplies:

Manicure supplies	Non-acetone polish remover
Acrylic liquid	Nail primer and applicator brush
Clear acrylic powder	
Sable nail brush	Nail sanitation brush
Nail tips	Three small containers (for liquid and powders)
Nail glue	
Acrylic nail file (coarse and medium)	Paper towels
	Manicuring implements
Nail buffer, emery block, swiss file	Acrylic nippers
	Duster brush
Orangewood stick	Oil or cream
Acetone	

FIGURE 7-1
Push back cuticle and roughen the nail bed.

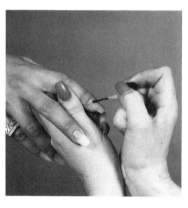

FIGURE 7-2
Dip the brush into clear powder and rotate to form an acrylic ball on the tip of brush.

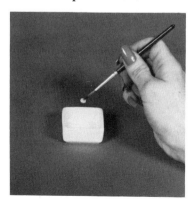

2. Follow pre-service rules.

3. Push back cuticle and lightly roughen nail bed (Figure 7-1).

4. Prime the nail bed with primer. Be careful not to get primer on cuticles or lunula (always use primer sparingly). If tip extensions are being used, be careful to only get primer on the natural nail, not on the tip.

5. Pour liquid into small dish and clear powder into another small dish.

6. Dip brush into liquid and remove the excess liquid by wiping brush on side of dish. Too much liquid makes it runny and not enough will make it too dry.

7. Dip the tip of brush into clear powder and rotate slightly, forming a ball of acrylic on tip of brush (Figure 7-2). Do not let acrylic get jammed into bristles of brush. Use brush only to apply acrylic to nail.

8. Place ball of acrylic on center of nail bed by touching nail with acrylic and turning the brush slightly (Figures 7-3 and 7-4). Wipe brush and dip into liquid; remove excess liquid by wiping brush on inside edge of dish.

FIGURE 7-3
Touch the nail with acrylic.

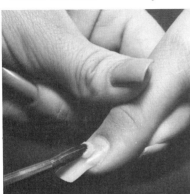

FIGURE 7-4
Turn brush slightly on nail.

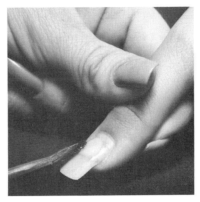

FIGURE 7-5
Blend acrylic into nail bed.

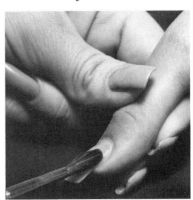

9. Hold brush at an angle so you can use flat part of the tip to *gently pat* the back center edge of acrylic making it blend into base of nail bed (Figure 7-5). Pat sides to blend while pressing acrylic slightly forward.

10. Form a second ball of acrylic and place on the tip (Figure 7-6). Use the same pat method to cover the end of tip.

11. Check nail from all angles to be sure acrylic covers the nail and tip evenly (Figure 7-7).

12. Smooth surface with brush; if needed you can add more acrylic a little at a time to even thickness of nail.

FIGURE 7-6
Form a second acrylic ball
and place it on the tip and
pat down.

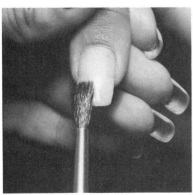

FIGURE 7-7
Check the nail to be sure tip
covers evenly.

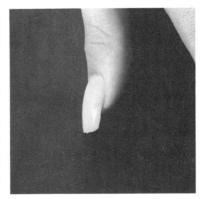

FIGURE 7-8
If thickness varies, add a little
more acrylic as needed.

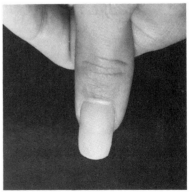

13. Put acrylic away so it doesn't get contaminated.

14. Always avoid cuticle. Use orangewood stick to remove any acrylic from cuticle before it dries.

15. Use nail file and shape the sides and surface of acrylic. Be sure to taper acrylic at the base of nail bed and at the tip. Check the shape of nail from all directions: both side views, front view, and back side. (See the section on filing techniques.)

16. Use buffer to smooth the nail surface. Use dark or roughest side first. Then use lighter or smoother side to finish. Oil at the end of buffing helps smooth nail and condition cuticles (Figures 7-9 and 7-10).

17. Continue on to next service: manicure, polish, or nail art (Figure 7-11).

FIGURE 7-9
Use the buffer to smooth the nail surface.

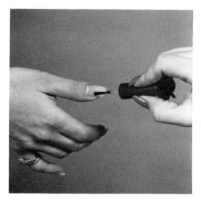

FIGURE 7-10
Use oil for a smooth finish.

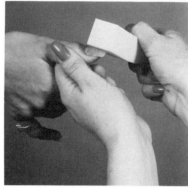

FIGURE 7-11
Continue on to the next service.

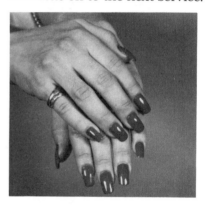

Points to Remember

1. Be sure nail bed is clean and dry before applying acrylic.
2. If using tips, be sure they are properly applied and shaped.
3. Never use too much primer.
4. Do not let primer touch skin. If it does, wash immediately to prevent burning.
5. Hold brush at an angle, using the flat part to shape acrylic.
6. Do not let acrylic dry on brush; keep it clean.
7. Only use the brush to apply and shape acrylic. It is not to be used like a paint brush; only the liquid should saturate the brush.
8. Do not cover the lunula.
9. Do not get acrylic in nail grooves.
10. Do not apply too thickly; too much filing can bruise the nail bed.

11. Support free edge when filing to avoid excess movement of nail bed and prevent discomfort.
12. Bevel end of nails for a natural look.
13. Buff nails until shiny for maximum results.

Sculptured Nails

Sculptured nails are made by a process of building the free edge with acrylic. A nail form is placed under the free edge and fits snugly against the underside of nail. When the form is properly in place, acrylic is applied in the shape of a nail. More acrylic is used to cover the nail bed and the new extension just made. Remember not to make the extension thick. If it is too thick, when the second layer is applied the nail will be too thick. When making the extended part of the nail, white powder is used instead of clear. The white looks natural instead of having a transparent nail. Because the natural grows with the acrylic the natural free edge remains next to the white extension as it grows away from the finger. This is why when doing fill-ins the white powder is not needed. Through the fill-in process clients can eventually grow their own nails and, little by little, file the sculptured extension away. Acrylic is still needed to add strength to the natural nail.

Procedure for Applying Sculptured Nails

1. Take out all acrylic supplies plus sculptured nail forms and white acrylic powder.
2. Follow pre-service rules.
3. Remove old nail polish and clean nails. Gently push back cuticles with cuticle pusher. Cut and file nails so they are even.
4. File the corners of nails round so the nail forms fit properly. Do not file into nail groove (Figure 7-12).
5. Dust powder off nail with duster brush.
6. Sanitize nails with disinfectant and let dry.

FIGURE 7-12
File corners of the nail round so the nail forms fit properly.

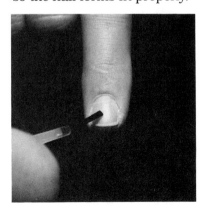

FIGURE 7-13
After the nails are sanitized, apply the primer carefully.

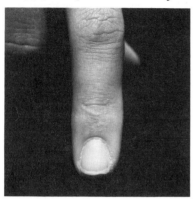

7. Apply primer to natural nail. Use sparingly and avoid the lunula and cuticle. Let dry (Figure 7-13).

8. Apply nail form under free edge.

   A. If using a reuseable nail form, pre-shape it close to the size of the finger being applied to. Slide the form under free edge and hold it against underside of nail. Press the form gently at the sides on end of finger. If there is a gap between the nail and form do not apply acrylic. Pull the front of form up while holding the sides. Do not wrap the ends of form around finger; this can make the front of form to tilt down and separate from nail. Press the sides only and keep up the form end.

   B. If using a disposable nail form with an adhesive backing, you can trim the sides of form making it less clumsy to handle (Figure 7-14). The tabs at end of form can also be trimmed to keep out of way if they don't stay stuck to finger. Do the trimming before you remove it from the backing so it won't stick to your fingers.

   Apply by telling client to hold finger out. Secure form from very edge of sides with first finger and thumb. To hold form bend first finger and use side of fingertip pressed to outer edge of thumb (Figure 7-15). By bending the finger, it is out of the way. Slide the form under the free edge and press the sides of form with thumbs

FIGURE 7-14
Trim the form if necessary.

FIGURE 7-15
To hold form, bend first finger and use the side of fingertip pressed to outer edge of thumb.

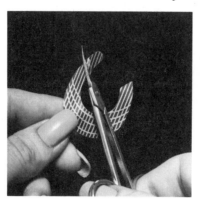

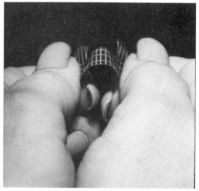

(Figure 7-16); hold with thumbs and pull first fingers down (Figure 7-17). Press form to sides of finger with thumbs and release. If form bends down or there is a space between nail and form, pull the tabs down and back (Figure 7-18). Then press the sides. Sometimes it is necessary to hold form in place while applying acrylic.

FIGURE 7-16
Slide the form under the free edge and press sides of form with thumb.

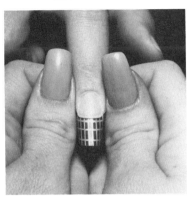

FIGURE 7-17
Hold the form at the sides to keep the shape.

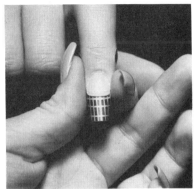

FIGURE 7-18
Check to see there is no space between nail and form.

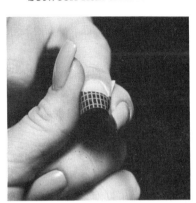

9. Pour liquid, clear powder and white powder into 3 separate containers.

10. Dip brush into liquid and wipe excess off on inside edge of container.

11. Dip tip of brush in white powder and rotate brush forming a ball on the end of brush. Do not let acrylic get jammed into the bristles of the brush. Use brush only to apply acrylic to the nail.

12. Place the white ball of acrylic on the edge of the free edge and nail form. Do not get it on natural nail, just on the form (Figure 7-19).

13. Hold brush at an angle so you can use flat part of brush tip to gently pat the acrylic (Figure 7-20). Shape the end of nail tip leaving the base of nail free of white acrylic (Figures

FIGURE 7-19
Place the white ball of acrylic on the free edge and nail form.

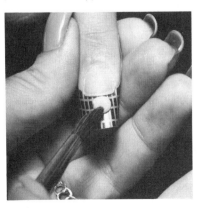

FIGURE 7-20
Hold brush at an angle.

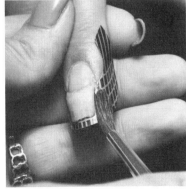

FIGURE 7-21
Shape the tip like the natural nail.

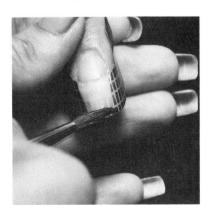

7-21, 7-22, and 7-23). Make this part thin and shaped like a natural nail; the better the shape, the less filing is needed.

FIGURE 7-22
Use the flat part of brush to shape the nail.

FIGURE 7-23
Keep white off the nail bed and give a natural curve to the free edge.

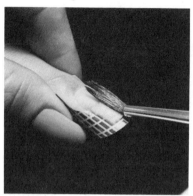

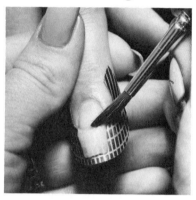

14. Using clear powder, form a ball on the end of brush and apply to base of nail blending acrylic into nail bed (Figure 7-24). Do not get on lunula or in nail grooves. Press acrylic evenly over the base of nail (Figure 7-25).

FIGURE 7-24
Form a ball with clear powder and apply to nail base.

FIGURE 7-25
Press acrylic evenly over nail base.

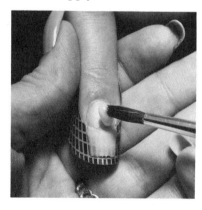

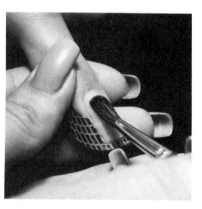

15. Again with clear acrylic, avoiding cuticle and lunula, cover the rest of the nail and tip (Figure 7-26), blending base of nail and extending over white extension, thicker at the breaking point for a stronger nail but not too thick; this also gives it a nice curve (Figure 7-27). Make sure acrylic is even by looking at nail from all angles (Figure 7-28).

16. Put acrylic away to prevent contamination.

FIGURE 7-26
Cover the rest of nail and tip
with acrylic.

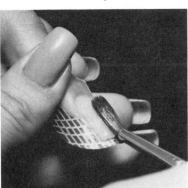

FIGURE 7-27
Make sure breaking point
is strong.

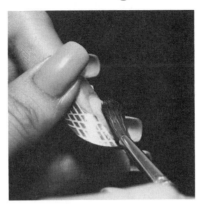

FIGURE 7-28
Check evenness of acrylic.

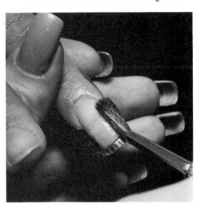

17. Allow nails to dry thoroughly (Figure 7-29); then tap nail with orangewood stick or file (Figure 7-30). If you hear a loud tapping sound it tells you the nail is dry; remove forms by pulling down and out carefully (Figures 7-31 and 7-32).

FIGURE 7-29
Allow nails to dry thoroughly.

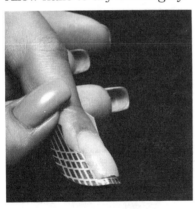

FIGURE 7-30
Tap nail to see if nail is dry.

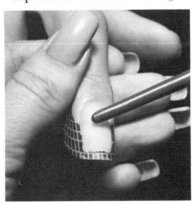

FIGURE 7-31
Carefully remove form from
sides of finger.

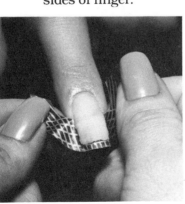

FIGURE 7-32
Gently pull form
from nail.

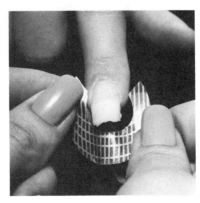

18. File end of nails to desired shape (Figures 7-33 and 7-34). Round, oval or square.

FIGURE 7-34
Next, file ridge on
the other side.

FIGURE 7-33
File ridge on one side.

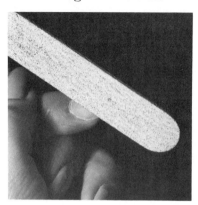
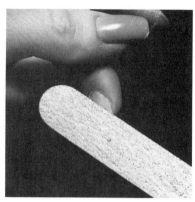

19. File top of nail (Figure 7-35), shaping sides and tapering toward the cuticle and tip (Figure 7-36). (See the section on filing techniques.)

FIGURE 7-36
Taper the nail toward the cuticle
and tip.

FIGURE 7-35
File nail end to desired shape.

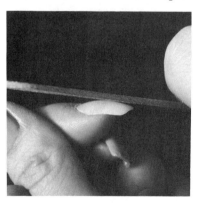
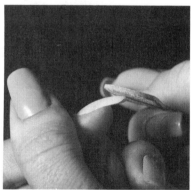

20. Buff nails with oil until smooth and shiny (Figure 7-37).

21. Continue onto next service: manicure, polish, or nail art (Figure 7-38).

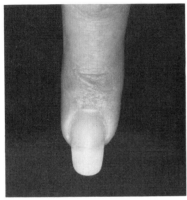

FIGURE 7-37
Buff nails with oil until
smooth.

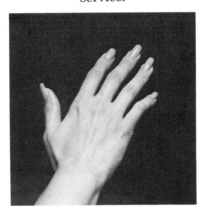

FIGURE 7-38
Continue on to the next
service.

Points to Remember

1. Don't get acrylic in the nail groove or on the moon.

2. When making the white tip do not make it too thick. Remember when you add the clear polish, it gets even thicker.

3. Be sure each nail has a nice curve by holding the form in the correct position while shaping the nail.

4. Make sure the shape of each nail matches; be consistent in your work.

5. Don't make nails too thick to cut down on filing time; try to make the nail as close to the desired end as possible.

6. When shaping the nail be sure the surface maintains the natural curve and is not left flat on top.

7. Be sure to buff the entire nail smooth; pay attention to the sides and the base for a natural look.

CHAPTER 8

Using Gels with and Without Light

INTRODUCTION

Working with gels presents a choice. There are light products with ultraviolet bonding. Directions may vary with each system. The other choice is to use a no-light gel. Nails are coated and bonded quickly after being sprayed. The latter gel is easy to use for patching and reshaping nails.

Light Nails or Ultraviolet Gel Bonding

There are many light nail products on the market. Each one has its own system and instructions. It is important to follow the instructions according to the system you are using.

A good system will have gel that doesn't run, is self-leveling, looks natural, and will not turn yellow. When properly used, it should bond to the nail tightly and will not lift off. This method of nail wrapping is fast and easy.

The following are basic instructions to be combined with the instructions in your kit.

Procedure for Using Gels with Light Bonding

1. Take out the following supplies:

Light nail ultraviolet lamp	Orangewood stick
Gels for lamp used	Paper towel
Brushes	Nail clean solution
Pre-nail prep	Soft file
Primer	Emery block
Nail tips or sculptured nail forms	Three-way buffer
Glue	Duster brush

2. Follow pre-service rules.
3. File free edge of natural nail to match the shape of nail tip being used. If making sculptured nails file corners round so nail form will fit snug.
4. Use a medium buffer to remove all shine from the nail bed. Pay close attention to the sides. Be sure there is no cuticle stuck to nail bed by gently pushing back with cuticle pusher.
5. Apply pre-nail preparation to sanitize nails.
6. Size all ten nail tips and apply. (See the section on nail tipping.)
7. Trim all ten nails and file one hand.
8. Dust nail tips with duster brush.
9. Apply nail primer sparingly, being sure to avoid cuticle and nail tip (Figure 8-1).

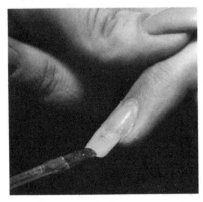

FIGURE 8-1
Apply nail primer sparingly.

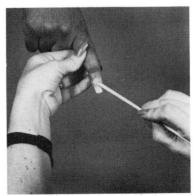

FIGURE 8-2
Adjust the amount of gel to the size of the nail.

10. Do four nails, leaving thumb for last. Use a gel brush and apply sufficient amount to cover nail. The amount of gel depends on the size of nail to be covered (Figure 8-2). If too

much gel is applied it will slide into the cuticle. Find a good medium, not too much or too little. The less pressure used with the brush, the thicker it will be; the more pressure used, the thinner it will be. Apply gel to base of nail just above the moon (don't touch cuticle). Using the tip of the brush, gently push gel back and lightly pull brush down the nail on each side and then down the center. Avoid lifting brush completely out of gel until you are at the end of nail tip to avoid air bubbles. Don't pat. If making a sculptured nail, use same method over nail form.

11. Place the four nails under the lamp. Tell client to remove fingers if any heat or pinch sensation occurs on their nail bed. If this happens, start time over again. The time under lamp depends on the instruction for your system.

12. File the other nail tips on second hand. If second coat is called for, you can apply it when timer goes off and then continue to file the other nails.

13. Apply gel to the four remaining fingers and place them under the lamp for amount of time required.

14. Apply gel to the thumbs last and place under the lamp (Figure 8-3). When all ten nails are cured, a sticky film remains on the surface; remove the film with nail cleaner provided with nail system.

15. Use a soft file to smooth the surface of nails. Shape the free edge to perfection.

16. Use an emery block to buff nails and finish with a three-way buffer to a great shine (Figure 8-4).

17. Give manicure and polish.

FIGURE 8-3
Apply gel to the thumb and place under lamp.

FIGURE 8-4
Use an emery block to buff nails to a good shine.

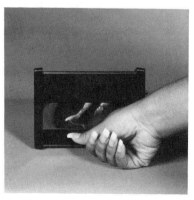

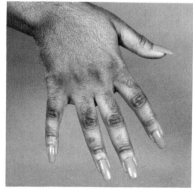

Points to Remember

1. When nails are under the lamp be sure all sides are exposed to the light. Some clients have very curved nail beds and may need to turn nails to one side and then the other to be absolutely sure that both sides are cured. This requires extra time under the lamp because each side must be cured for the full amount of time to be sure gel is set on the edge of nail grooves.
2. This product cannot be removed with acetone. Follow instructions from manufacture of products.
3. Tell client if heat sensation occurs to remove their hand from under the lamp.
4. Follow instructions for your gel system.

No-Light Gel Nails

The no-light gel nail system is very fast and easy. The nail is coated with a thick gel and set with an activator spray that hardens the gel almost instantly and bonds it to the nail.

The gel is also easy to use for patching and reshaping nails. It is fast and very popular with clients. Avoid getting this product on the lunula in the nail grooves or anywhere except where it belongs. When sprayed it hardens and sticks.

Proper use is crucial if maximum results are expected. Every system is similar but also slightly different in the procedure of preparing the nail and setting the gel.

Tell the client of the possibilities involved, such as chemical burning, especially if there is damage to the nail bed or client sensitivity.

Procedure for No-Light Gel Nails

1. Take out the following supplies:

No-light gel system kit	Files
No-light gel	Buffers
Gel activator spray	Orangewood stick
Nail preparation/sanitation method	Duster brush

2. Follow pre-service rules.
3. Lightly roughen nail with light to medium grade file. If applying nail tips do so now.

4. Use duster brush to remove dust from nail bed and free edge.

5. Sanitize the nails and let dry.

6. Squeeze the amount needed to evenly cover the entire nail (except the lunula) to the center of nail (Figure 8-5). Quickly use orangewood stick to spread gel over nail very evenly (Figure 8-6). Gel will level and smooth itself out after you

FIGURE 8-5
Squeeze gel needed to cover entire nail except lunula.

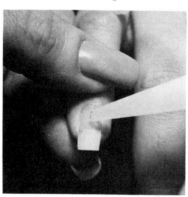

FIGURE 8-6
Use an orangewood stick to spread the gel.

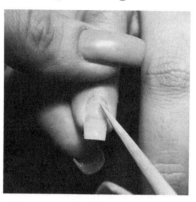

spread it around as evenly as possible. A nail that is slightly crooked, dipped, or narrow on the end can be reshaped with gel by adding extra gel to the needed area after the first coat is set. Sometimes a second coat is needed. If any gel runs into the nail groove or gets on the lunula it must be removed completely with an orangewood stick before it is set with the activator spray (Figure 8-7).

7. When nail is covered perfectly, follow the instructions for the system being used to see how far to hold the spray from nail. Spray nail to set gel (Figure 8-8).

FIGURE 8-7
Clean gel from nail groove and lunula.

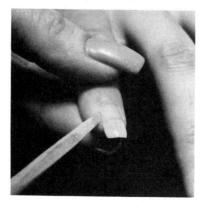

FIGURE 8-8
Follow distance directions for spraying nail.

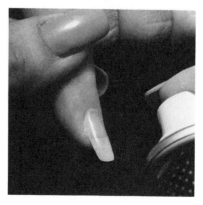

8. After coating all nails, file them lightly. If you apply gel right, very little filing should be needed.
9. Buff nails to remove any scratches (Figure 8-9).
10. Give next desired service.

FIGURE 8-9
After buffing, give the next desired service.

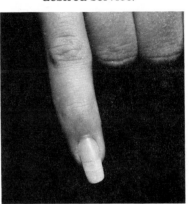

Points to Remember

1. Apply gel on a clean and prepared nail.
2. Be sure nail grooves are free of gel before spraying. Do not apply too much gel at one time.
3. Hold spray at a distance according to instructions.
4. Do not overfile.

Removal of No-Light Gel

The product can be soaked in acetone to remove. Do not pry away from nail to avoid damage to natural nail.

Maintenance for No-Light Gel Nails

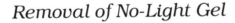

To do a maintenance manicure with gel instead of glue, cover the entire nail. Do not make it too thick at the end of the nail; use only where it is needed. Fill-ins are not needed because you are filling in each time you do a maintenance manicure with the gel.

CHAPTER 9

Patches and Repairs

INTRODUCTION

Unfortunately sometimes damage occurs to nails causing wraps to chip, crack, lift away from nail bed, or a nail can break off completely at the breaking point. If a nail or wrap is very damaged sometimes it's better to completely remove it and apply a new wrap with or without an extension. If it is only partially damaged then usually it can be patched or repaired. Slightly different techniques are used for different wrap types. For fiberglass patching use the same methods as for silk and linen; however with fiberglass you use an activator rather than glue. Acrylic, sculptured, light gel, and cotton patching, as well as crack repair, are explained. The objective is the same for all types. Patch or repair it like new.

Silk, Linen, and Fiberglass Patching

A nail wrap can be easily patched when it chips at the edges or separates from the free edge. If the side is worn away or chipped off, it can be fixed, even if the natural nail or extension cracks at breaking point.

Procedure for Patching Silk, Linen, and Fiberglass Wraps

1. Take out the following supplies:
   Manicure supplies
   Silk, linen, or fiberglass supplies

2. Follow pre-service rules.

3. Remove old nail polish and clean the nail. Gently push back cuticles. (If repairing a cracked nail, refer to the section on cracked nails now. If making a regular patch continue on.)

4. Carefully clip away loose wrap from damaged area. Do not pull or tear wrap off; clip it gently so you do not loosen the wrap more. Don't dig on the natural nail.

5. Use a medium grade file to smooth clipped area and lightly file the rest of the wrap removing any loose wrap from edges and discoloration from old polish.

6. Dust the nail with duster brush to remove filing dust.

7. Sanitize nails with disinfectant. Let dry. (If fixing a side refer to the section on fixing sides now. If making a regular patch continue on.)

8. Prepare fabric by cutting a small strip, wide enough to cover the area to be patched and long enough to hold.

9. Apply one drop of glue directly on the end of fabric and set glued fabric on area to be patched. Do not let fabric touch cuticle or skin by holding the end of fabric toward the center of the nail.

10. Use the orangewood stick or plastic to press fabric in place. Then cut the excess fabric off with small scissors.

11. Let dry or spray lightly with instant glue setter at least six inches away from nail.

12. File the patch lightly until smooth.

13. Cover the entire nail wrap with glue. Spread glue evenly over nail with the orangewood stick.

14. Turn palm up and use an orangewood stick to apply glue to edges of wrap. Be sure all edges are glued together.

Acrylic, Sculptured Nail, and Light Gel Patching

Use the fill-in technique for these wraps; only fill in the area to be patched after preparing the nail. When patching the side or end of a nail nip away loose wrap, then file until it is even and smooth. Glue remaining wrap to secure it to the nail and fill in the area using whatever patching product is needed.

Repairing Cracked Nails

1. To repair a crack file the entire wrap until it is as thin as you can get it without removing it completely.
2. Follow the rest of patching instructions from step 5.
3. After patching the crack, wrap the entire nail by following wrapping techniques (see Chapter 6).

Fixing Sides with Fabric

Fabric patching techniques can be used to repair or reshape a worn side.

Procedure for Fixing Sides with Fabric

1. Use fabric wrapping supplies.
2. To fix the side of nail use a strip of fabric long enough to cover length of nail and hold onto it with your fingers (Figure 9-1).
3. Apply a drop of glue to end of fabric and place it on the side of nail leaving an overlap to make new side to nail (Figure 9-2).

FIGURE 9-1
Fabric should cover the length of nail.

FIGURE 9-2
Apply glue to end of fabric and place it on the side of the nail.

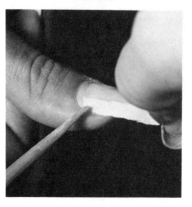
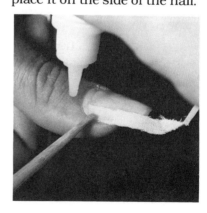

4. Press fabric onto nail with an orangewood stick or plastic (Figures 9-3 and 9-4).
5. Cut excess fabric from nail and glue (Figure 9-5).

| **FIGURE 9-3** | **FIGURE 9-4** | **FIGURE 9-5** |
| Use an orangewood stick to smooth out the fabric. | Plastic can also be used to press down fabric. | Cut excess fabric and glue. |

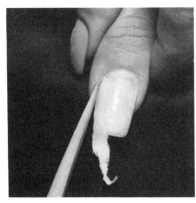

FIGURE 9-3
Use an orangewood stick to smooth out the fabric.

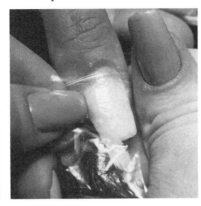

FIGURE 9-4
Plastic can also be used to press down fabric.

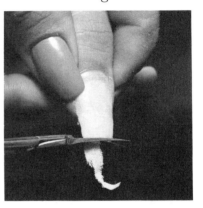

FIGURE 9-5
Cut excess fabric and glue.

6. Buff nail and coat again with glue; then buff and give next service.

Extending the Free Edge with Fabric

The free edge can be extended using the same technique used for fixing sides. The difference is you put the fabric across the end of nail letting it overlap. Trim the fabric to the desired length and glue. Several layers can be used to make it stronger. It is not recommended to make extensions too long.

Points to Remember

1. Keep the cuticle and nail groove clean.
2. Check underside edges to be sure it is glued securely.
3. Do not overfile and remove patch.
4. If nail is badly damaged it is better to soak the nail clean and start fresh.

Cotton Patch

The cotton patch method is really great for repairing a cracked nail before you wrap it for added strength.

The natural nail can be repaired, then wrapped with silk or coated with any other clear wrapping technique to make it very natural looking and strong.

A cotton patch is useful in many cases, but always remember that a badly broken nail tip should be removed first. Then fix the crack in the natural nail before applying a new tip. This will ensure a better patch, especially if the crack is right in the breaking point.

Procedure for Cotton Patch

1. Take out the following supplies:

Cotton   Nail file (medium grade and soft grade)
Nail glue   Buffers

2. Follow pre-service rules.

3. Clean break or crack in nail. If there is a nail tip on the nail and it is cracked as well as the natural nail, then you must carefully soak the nail until it is completely clean. (Figure 9-6).

4. Lightly buff the nail with coarse buffer.

5. Dust with duster brush.

6. Pull a small section of cotton partially apart while carefully twisting center of cotton until you have made a thin string in the center.

7. Hold each side of string about one inch apart and slide it into the crack as far to the end of break as possible (Figure 9-7).

FIGURE 9-6
Crack or break in nail should be cleaned.

FIGURE 9-7
Slide thin cotton string into the crack as far to the end as possible.

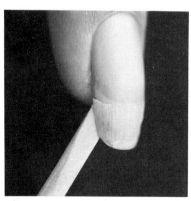
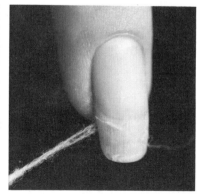

8. Gently pull the bottom section of string out to the edge of the nail. Do not pull too hard or it might break. Hold onto the end of the string to keep it smooth.

9. Apply glue to the top of nail on crack; before it dries, gently tug on the bottom piece of cotton string and wrap it over the top of crack (Figure 9-8).

10. Twist the two pieces together on top of nail and glue again (Figure 9-9).

FIGURE 9-8
Fold cotton string over top of nail, covering the crack.

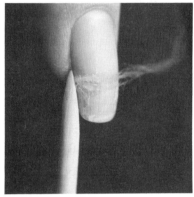

FIGURE 9-9
After twisting and gluing, cut cotton off the top of nail.

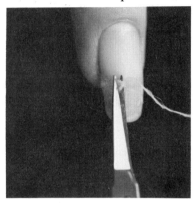

11. Clip off extra cotton and lightly file the bump smooth (Figure 9-10).

12. Glue area again and buff.

13. If patch sticks out at the side file it just a tiny bit and glue it again.

14. Wrap nail or apply a tip and wrap, whichever is desired.

FIGURE 9-10
Lightly file the bump until it is smooth.

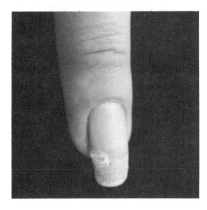

FIGURE 9-11
The stick points to where crack was in the nail.

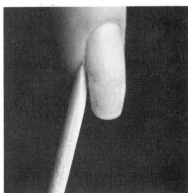

Points to Remember

1. Clean nail thoroughly before patching.
2. Do not file the edge of patch too much or it will not hold.
3. Cover area with glue after each filing.
4. Remove broken wrap or nail tip completely or it will not hold very long.
5. Be sure nail groove and underside of nail are not glued or client will pick at it and weaken patch or break it again.

Fixing a Break on the Nail Bed

Repairing a badly broken nail that is below the breaking point usually hurts a little. Take great care in avoiding being rough; remember this is an injury to the nail bed. If the nail is too tender to touch or is bleeding, do not glue it. Hold the nail in place and cut the nail as short as the client allows. This will minimize movement of nail tip. Sanitize the nail and, while holding it straight, place a band-aid carefully around the nail. Tell the client to keep it clean. After a day or two you can patch the break or put on a tip and wrap. The nail will still be tender so be gentle, especially before you glue the crack: Do not remove polish until the nail is glued.

Procedure for Fixing a Break on the Nail Bed

1. Take out all supplies needed for wrap being used. This depends on the kind of wrap already on the nail.
2. First remove the bandaid; cut with scissors so it doesn't pull nail. The skin is still attached to the nail so be very careful.
3. Warn the client the nail might hurt for a few seconds.
4. Adjust the nail so it is in place and hold it there gently and press it together.
5. Apply a drop of glue to each side of the nail at the break. With an orangewood stick, spread glue over the top of nail.
6. After glue dries clip the nail as short as possible, without making it too short and out of place with the others. This helps to avoid banging or hitting the nail until it grows.
7. Remove nail polish and gently file off the remaining polish under the glue. Glue again lightly and let dry.

8. Very gently wrap the nail. If wrapping with a product that requires priming you must skip it this time on the broken nail to avoid getting it in the break. Be sure to sanitize the nail. Although this might sting a little, it will help prevent infection.

Points to Remember

1. Be careful not to hurt the client.
2. Do not put glue into the crack; hold the nail together and spread glue over the top.
3. Trim nail shorter so it is less likely to be bumped and get sore.
4. Try not to move the nail too much.
5. File gently.
6. Do not overglue.

CHAPTER 10

Fill-Ins

INTRODUCTION

The proper care of artificial nails or nail wraps is very important. Clients must be aware of the problems that arise with improper maintenance.

As the nail grows forward, a broad space develops between the product and cuticle. To keep the nail strong, a balance must be maintained. To do this, a fill-in is needed, adding the product used to fill-in the space that has developed from the nail growth. This not only strengthens the nail near the breaking point, but also adds weight to the base of the nail which balances the weight of the whole nail making it stronger. This prevents lifting of the product at the base of the nail bed.

Your client should be told to get fill-ins according to individual need. If the nails grow fast, a fill-in should be done every two or three weeks. Glue manicures once a week extremely extends the life of a wrap; now and then a patch may be needed.

If the nails grow slowly, once a month might be enough. A good way to determine the length of time between fill-ins is to check the nail growth in two weeks. If it has grown so much that the wrap is near the breaking point, a fill-in is needed. If not, take in mind how much the nail grew and determine how much more time might be needed for the nail to grow out. Keep in mind the length of your client's nail bed also—the longer the nail bed, the longer the space can be between product and cuticle before the nail becomes weak.

Procedure for Linen, Silk, and Fiberglass Fill-Ins

1. Take out the following supplies:

   Manicuring implements and supplies

   Linen or silk

   Fast-drying nail glue

   Disinfectant

   Coarse and medium files

   Medium and fine buffers

   Orangewood stick

   Dust Brush

   Straight scissors

2. Remove nail polish.

3. Check nails for cracks or lifting of product.

4. Using acrylic nippers, carefully clip away loose product if any. Do not pry or dig into the nail bed. This will cause damage to the natural nail (be careful of flying pieces of product).

5. Using a coarse file on the existing wrap, smooth the area at the fill-in line. Then file over the surface of the rest of wrap to obtain a fresh surface.

6. Gently buff the exposed part of nail bed (avoid the lunula).

7. Remove any dust or particles with the duster brush.

8. Apply disinfectant protection only *to natural nail*. Let dry.

9. Wrap area to be filled in using fabric wrap techniques. (See the section on linen and silk wraps.)

10. Take scissors and trim precisely to the edge of nail at sides; be sure there is no fabric touching cuticle. Cut end off halfway down nail or at least $\frac{1}{4}$ inch past old wrap.

11. Holding the finger down so the free edge is slanted toward the table, apply nail glue over the *entire* nail. Avoid getting glue on the cuticle (holding nail slanting down will avoid glue from running into the cuticle). Let dry. An instant glue setter can be used to speed up drying time.

12. Using a medium file, smooth the wrap by holding the file flat (see the section on filing techniques).

13. Apply the final coat of nail glue on entire nail. Use an orangewood stick to spread the glue evenly over the nail. Be sure to check the edges and underside of nail to see that all is secure and neat.

14. Buff nails first with a medium buffer, then with a fine buffer until perfectly smooth.

15. Give manicure and polish.

Points to Remember

1. Remove loose or lifting area, if any.
2. Be sure remaining wrap is secure.
3. Blend new wrap with rest of nail.
4. Check end of nails if shortened; if thick you can bevel the end for a natural look.
5. Book next appointment.

Procedure for Acrylic Fill-Ins

1. Take out the following supplies:

   Manicuring implements and   Disinfectant
      supplies   Primer
   Liquid   Nail files and buffers
   Clear powder   Orangewood stick
   Sable brush

2. Remove polish.
3. With nippers, carefully clip away loose acrylic, if any. (Do not dig into nail bed. Be careful of flying acrylic chips.)
4. File the ridge smooth and gently roughen exposed part of nail bed. Lightly file away any discoloration on the rest of the nail.
5. Remove any dust or powder.
6. Disinfect nail and let dry.
7. Prime nails; do not put primer on acrylic, only the exposed natural nail.
8. Dip brush in liquid container and wipe excess liquid on the side of the container.
9. Dip brush in clear powder and rotate, forming a small ball on the end of the brush.
10. Apply ball on exposed nail, making sure the acrylic does not get on the cuticle. (There is no need to put acrylic over entire nail—only where it is needed to fill-in).
11. Check entire nail to make sure the acrylic evenly covers all of the nail. Add more acrylic where needed. Let dry.
12. File nail to smooth out the filled area. Bevel the end of nail and shorten at this time, if desired, with file.
13. Buff, give manicure, and polish.

Points to Remember

1. Remove any lifting acrylic with nippers.
2. File the acrylic surface till it is clean and reshape before adding more acrylic for fill-in.
3. Do not get too close to lunula.
4. Keep nail grooves clean.
5. Nail should look good as new when done.

Procedure for Light and No-Light Gel Fill-Ins

1. Take out the following supplies:

Manicuring implements and supplies	Glue
	Orangewood stick
Gels (lamp if using light-gel)	Paper towel
Brushes	Nail cleaning solution
Pre-nail prep	Soft file
Primer	Emery block
Nail tips or sculptured nail form	Three-way buffer
	Duster brush

2. Remove nail polish and push back cuticles.
3. Use medium coarse file and file the surface of all nails to remove all ridges and discolored areas. Any discoloration indicates lifting of product and should be carefully removed with file or nippers.
4. Remove dust with duster brush.
5. Prime nails.
6. Apply gel to nails in the same manner as when doing a full set. Pay attention to the base of the nail bed and don't make the free edge too thick.
7. Check the breaking point. Add more gel if needed; then cure and remove sticky film.
8. Complete as you would a full set.
9. Manicure and polish.

Points to Remember

1. Follow directions of system being used.
2. Be sure nail is free of loose products.
3. Do not cover lunula.
4. Keep nail grooves clean.

CHAPTER 11

Removal
Techniques

INTRODUCTION

Removing tips or wraps of every kind is necessary sometimes—if a nail breaks or is damaged badly, or if a client is sensitive to nail product and has a bad reaction. Maybe a client would like to change services from fiberglass to acrylic nails for greater strength, or change the shape of the nail surface for cosmetic reasons. For whatever reason you need to remove the nail product, it must be done with one foremost concern: Do not damage the natural nail. Do not dig in nail grooves or in lunula. Always treat the nail bed gently and remove the nail product properly.

There are several methods of removing different products. Always follow manufacturer directions if a special product or procedure is required. The removal process starts by trimming any excess tip or loose wrap from nails; then soaking nails in a nail product remover. There are many kinds of removal products available from pure acetone, tip remover, glue remover, gel remover, and so on. Most products have an acetone base. Acetone is great for removing most wraps but is very drying and should not be overused. The best way to find a removal product is to try whatever you can and use what works best for you. Keep in mind the cost of fancy aromatic removers; they may not work as well as polish remover or pure acetone.

Removal of Fabric and Fiberglass Wraps

If a client is wearing a fabric wrap with extensions, the tips must be cut off even with the natural nail. This gives less to soak off. If the wrap is protecting the natural nail, then just gently nip away any loose wrap before soaking.

Procedure for Removal of Linen, Silk, and Fiberglass Wraps

1. Take out the following supplies:

    Small glass bowl or container   Orangewood stick
    Acetone or product remover   Coarse and medium files
    Manicure supplies   Paper towels
    Large clippers

2. Follow pre-service rules.
3. If wearing tip extensions, use large clippers and cut off even with natural nails (Figure 11-1).
4. Carefully nip off loose parts of wrap, if any.
5. If wrap is very thick use a coarse file to remove the bulk of wrap.
6. Check fingers to see what is needed (Figure 11-2).

FIGURE 11-1
Use large clippers to cut off tip extension even with the natural nail.

FIGURE 11-2
Check nails to see what is needed.

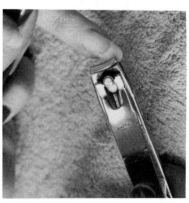

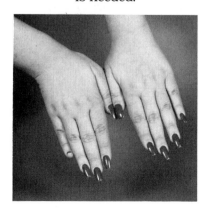

7. Pour removal solution into bowl deep enough to cover the top of nails. Place fingertips in bowl with nail bed facing up or at least straight up and down (Figure 11-3). If client curls fingers and puts the nail bed on bottom of dish it will take longer to soak. Any place the nail bed touches the bowl the remover is not. Be sure the fingers are in the right position to save time.

8. Let soak until the glue melts away. You can check by using the orangewood stick to gently scrape the nail (Figure 11-4).

FIGURE 11-3
Soak nail to remove old wrap.

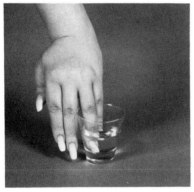

FIGURE 11-4
Use an orangewood stick to gently scrape wrap off the nail.

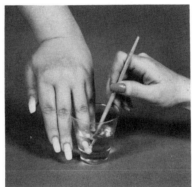

If it has soaked long enough the fabric should slide off the nail. If wrap is thick you can let it soak partially and rub the melting glue and wrap off with a medium coarse file and soak again. Repeat the process until the nail is almost clean. The last part of a thick wrap should be soaked, then rubbed with a paper towel.

FIGURE 11-5
After removal and buffing, give manicure or desired service.

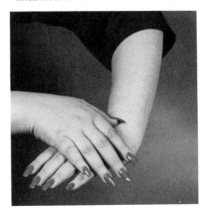

9. Buff nails lightly to remove any residue from glue or other product.

10. Give manicure or other desired nail service (Figure 11-5). If none is required, then condition cuticles and apply a base coat and top coat for some protection.

Removal of Acrylic Wraps

If the client has sculptured nails or acrylic tip extensions follow this procedure for removal.

Procedure for Removing Acrylic Wraps

1. Take out supplies for removing fabric and fiberglass wraps.
2. Follow pre-service rules.
3. If removing sculptured nails, acrylic or other product over tips then cut tips off with large clippers. To save the free edge of the natural nail do not cut tips.
4. Remove any loose product with nippers.
5. Pour remover in bowl and soak nails until the acrylic melts off the nail. You can see it get bumpy and thick when it melts. To speed up the process, carefully scrape with an orange-wood stick or wipe each nail with paper towel and quickly put back in remover to soak again.
6. Continue this process until acrylic is gone. It is faster to leave it in until it has all soaked off. When the nail is removed from the bowl it starts to harden again, so keep the fingers in bowl unless product is very thick and needs extra help in removing.

Removing Light and No-Light Gels

This product should be removed following directions from manufacturer of product used since these vary in procedure. Always remember to avoid damage to natural nail and cuticles. Products that are difficult to remove can damage the nail and you must decide if it is worth using.

Points to Remember

1. Keep top of nail beds exposed to remover for faster soaking.
2. File the bulk of the wrap off before soaking.
3. If removing tips, cut them off first; this keeps the time down and the mess.
4. Use paper towels to wipe melting product from nails; tissue or cotton is not strong or durable enough. Gauze pads are great but costly.
5. Clean under the nail as well as on top.
6. Do not scrape hard or dig on the nail bed to remove product.
7. When filing melted product be careful not to file through to natural nail.
8. Do not let client take nail or nails out of bowl to look. Tell them to soak until you remove them. This avoids a big mess and stops the slowing down of removing product. Condition cuticles after all other services are done.

CHAPTER 12

Polish and Nail Art

INTRODUCTION

After nails are shaped beautifully they deserve the best to finish the look. A natural look can be achieved by using a clear polish over most nails or white tips can be painted on for the unpolished "polished" look. Some prefer colored polish, from sheer and shiny to dark red enamel. Other ways to decorate nails are to apply different art mediums to the nails using them as tiny canvasses or in some cases long tiny canvasses. Simple designs with decorative nail tape or gems are used over polished nails. Real gold leaf is layered on the nails as is other items such as feathers, lace, snake skin, and hand painted pictures. Gold charms are pierced through the free edge and bolted on and entire gold nails are used to cover a nail. The ideas are endless and the combination of art mediums can create amazing results from spectacular to conservative with a splash of fun. The first thing to do is polish the nails to prepare a backdrop for most nail art. Let this dry completely with a top coat before starting to decorate the nails.

Polishing Technique

This is the finishing touch to all your work. After using all your talent to create beautiful nails you must finish with a perfect polish job. Some clients prefer a clear polish for the natural look but most want a colored polish of their choice. A perfect polish job is one that covers the entire nail and has no streaks or lumps. Also it should be close to the cuticle as possible without touching it. If it is applied too thick or if each coat is put on before the previous one has dried, it will not dry completely for a long time and will most likely get smudged before it dries. A top coat of clear polish protects the color from being scratched or rubbed off. Quick drying products help protect the polish surface until completely dry. Application of polish should be done on clean nails for best results and for longer wear. (See the section on removing polish.) It is a good idea to prepare client to walk out the door before you start, such as getting out keys or travel fare, paying the bill, or putting on coat if they can't sit to let the artwork dry.

Procedure for Polishing

1. Take out the following supplies:

   Base coat or ridge filler
   Nail polish (color of choice)
   Top coat
   Orangewood stick or corrector stick
   Quick dry (spray or brush on)

2. Hold client's finger firm at the side near the cuticle. Gently pull skin away from the cuticle and hold it back to avoid getting polish on it.
3. Gently push back the cuticle.
4. Apply a base coat by removing applicator brush from bottle and wipe once on the inside edge of bottle. Place the end of brush just below lunula and press down to spread bristles out creating a fan-like appearance to the end of bristles. At the same time, gently push polish up almost to the cuticle and then pull brush down the length of nail. Use the same technique to polish sides of nail. Make sure nail is covered completely and evenly.
5. Use an orangewood stick to remove polish from cuticle or skin if any.
6. Repeat steps 3 and 4 to each nail.
7. To each nail apply one coat of color in same manner as base coat application. Let dry one minute before applying the next coat. This layer does not have to be too close to the cuticle; for the second coat you must concentrate on getting close. Too much time is wasted removing mistakes twice.

8. Apply the second coat of color. After polishing each nail remove any polish from cuticle and nail grooves before polish dries and hardens.

9. The last step is to protect the color with one layer of top coat. Be sure the top coat covers completely and evenly on every nail.

10. Apply quick dry to polished fingers. If using a spray, hold it at least six inches from nails and spray lightly. If using a brush on quick dry, avoid brush marks in polish by placing saturated brush on edge of cuticle instead of on the nail. Brush down nail very lightly; use same method for the sides of nail.

Helpful Hints for Polishing

Extend pinky or ring finger on hand you are polishing with. Use this extension as a brace by placing it on client's hand or the table. Find the most comfortable position for you. The brace will help you be steady and reduce shaking for a neater job.

To remove excess polish from cuticle and nail groove without removing it from the nail is tricky. Try putting the tool of choice on the cuticle edge instead of on the nail, slightly rotate tool away from the nail to gently pull away, carefully press into the area to be cleaned while pulling skin back, and wipe polish off skin without touching the nail.

Points to Remember

1. Gently pull cuticle back at sides of nail to polish and remove mistakes.

2. Use the right amount of polish on the brush according to nail size.

3. Press base of brush down to spread bristles to make a clean line at base of nail.

4. Do not make base coat and first coat of color too thick to impede drying quickly.

5. Be sure to completely cover nail with second coat of color.

6. Remove mistakes on skin before polish dries.

7. Always use a top coat to seal and protect polish.

French Manicure

FIGURE 12-1
The French manicure has a
white tip on the free edge of
the nail.

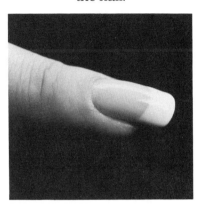

The french manicure is a special way of polishing the nail. A sheer or light pink color is used for the first color; then a white stripe is painted on the free edge of the nail (Figure 12-1). Make each white stripe the same width. After the white a sheer beige or pink tone is applied over the whole nail blending it all together. Some clients prefer a line that goes straight across and others like it to arch slightly with the natural nail shape. The french manicure is very popular and if done correctly enhances uneven nails to create an illusion that every nail is the same length, as well as clean and white.

Some variations of the french manicure are popular; try making a "V" shape or create a design. You can use different sheer colors for the top layer for a different look.

Procedure for a French Manicure

1. Take out the following supplies:

   French manicure kit or,
   (a) Base coat
   (b) Desired color of base (pink or natural tone)
   (c) White nail polish
   (d) Top color of choice (sheer pink or beige) or any other sheer color for a different look
   (e) Top coat

   Orangewood stick
   Nail polish remover

2. Give needed nail services including a manicure; stop before polishing the nails.
3. Apply base coat and let dry about two minutes.
4. Apply an even but not too thick coat of pink base color and let dry two minutes.
5. Shake bottle of white before using, and after about every other nail since it thickens quickly. If it seems sticky, it is better to throw the bottle away before it is completely empty rather than thin it or use it thick and sticky.
6. Hold client's finger so you can turn it easily. Make sure client is relaxed since you are going to turn the finger one way and paint the white strip in the other direction. In this way it is done in one swipe clear across the nail from one side of the free edge to the other. Continue in the same way on the other nail side, so each side is freshly colored with a

newly dipped brush and crossed in the middle to even itself out. Practice this procedure on yourself to get really good at it.

7. This step is crucial to making it last. Let the white strip dry for at least three to five minutes before applying the next coat. Explain to the client it is better to let the nails dry thoroughly before applying the finishing touches. You can start another client or confirm some appointments, or do something else. To sit there with the client seems like forever for both of you; be sure the client does not mess up the nails before letting them dry.

8. Apply the top color of choice; usually one coat is required if using a sheer beige or a light sheer pink. A very sheer color that is thinner like pearl, silver, or sheer opal might need two coats; let each coat dry between layers.

9. A protective top coat is the last layer and should be applied with great care in covering the nail evenly and completely.

10. If a client likes, a quick dry can help protect the service while letting the nails dry.

Points to Remember

1. Keep a steady hand while painting the white strip by extending the little finger on the hand that is holding the brush. Rest the extended finger on the other hand to brace yourself.

2. Do not make the white strip too thick or it won't dry.

3. Make each nail the same to make a perfect set of nails.

4. Let each layer of polish dry as much as possible between coats. A higher price is charged for the french manicure so a little more time to make it perfect is worthwhile. Save extra time by practicing and getting the polish done perfectly and quickly every time.

5. Try making your own special design.

6. Tell the client to apply another layer of top coat after a couple of days to freshen it and make it last longer.

Nail Gem Application

Nails can be beautifully enhanced using gem stones or rhinestones. One or more gems are placed on the nail in wet, clear polish. When the polish dries the gem stays stuck on the nail. One gem can be used to enhance a design made with another medium or several others. Also you can create the design with the gems. Use your imagination to create your own works of art.

Procedure for Applying Nail Gems

1. Take out the following supplies:

   Orangewood stick   Nail gems
   Clear top coat   Nail polish corrector

2. Polish nails in a regular manner by applying base coat, two coats of color, and one layer of top coat. Let dry completely.
3. Determine position of nail gem.
4. Use the very end of top coat brush and put one dot of top coat where gem will be placed.
5. Apply a small amount of top coat to the end of an orangewood stick.
6. Touch the top of gem with the wet end of the stick and pick gem up.
7. Press gem on to the dot of top coat on nail.
8. Repeat steps 1 through 5 until gem pattern is complete.
9. After all gems are in place, apply one layer of top coat over the entire nail and gems.
10. Let dry.
11. Use clean tip of nail polish corrector to carefully remove excess top coat from surface of gems so that they sparkle.
12. Let dry completely.

Points to Remember

1. Always apply a top coat and let it dry first to protect polish from mistakes.
2. Set gems on second layer or on spots of wet top coat.
3. Using an orangewood stick to gently push gems you can arrange or relocate them before polish dries.
4. When applying the top coat over finished design, use a little extra and apply slowly to avoid air bubbles.
5. Clean surface of gems after polish has dried or leave gems covered completely for more protection. They do not sparkle as much when covered with a top coat.

Nail Tape Application

The nail tape is used by removing the backing from tape and pressing the sticky side on to the nail. After the design is complete, clear nail polish is used to cover the tape sealing it under the polish and keeping it in place. The nail tape can be used with other design mediums to create unique nail art. Experiment with everything.

Procedure for Nail Tape

1. Take out the following supplies:

   Self-adhesive nail design tape   Sharp nippers
   Polish

2. Polish nails in a regular manner by applying base coat, two coats of color, and one layer of top coat. Let dry completely.
3. In one hand hold the end of tape; in the other hand, hold roll of tape (make sure not to touch the sticky back of the tape or it won't stick on nail).
4. Place tape on nail and cut the end (leave the ends long until pattern is complete).
5. Use an orangewood stick to firmly press tape down.
6. Trim all edges at once so they are even (Figure 12-2).
7. Apply top coat over tape. While top coat is drying, use an orangewood stick to gently press ends of tape down if they pop up.

FIGURE 12-2
Trim all edges at once so they are even.

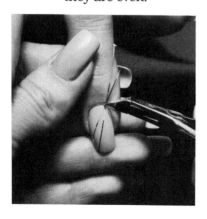

8. Check to see that all ends of tape are secure. Then apply last layer to top coat paying close attention to sides of nails and ends to tape (Figure 12-3).
9. Let dry completely.

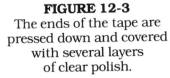

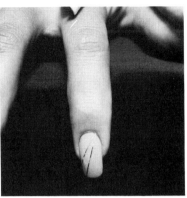

Points to Remember

1. Be sure top coat is completely dry before applying tape.
2. Trim all ends together ensuring that they are all even.
3. Do not touch the sticky back of tape.
4. A tiny drop of glue can be used to secure ends if they stick up.
5. Cover tape completely; several coats are needed to bury the tape under a top coat.
6. Apply top coat slowly to avoid air bubbles.

Nail Art Feathers

There are many beautiful feathers to make great designs with. Alone or combined with any other medium used on nails the feather is usually one of the most admired for its intriguing concept in nail art. The following instructions are basic for the application of a feather to a polished nail. You can use your imagination and create your own designs by using this technique in various ways. Experiment and have fun.

Feathers are applied to the nail with clear nail polish. Several layers of clear polish under and over the feather will bury it and seal it on to the nail. The feather can cover the entire nail or part of it.

Procedure for Nail Art Feathers

1. Take out the following supplies:

   Top coat   Orangewood stick
   Feathers   Tweezers
   Scissors

2. Polish nails with desired color and top coat. Let dry. If polish is wet, the color will mush through feather and make it look messy.

3. After nail is dry apply another coat of clear polish; while wet, set feather into clear polish (Figure 12-4).

4. Arrange with an orangewood stick to the desired position.

5. Apply clear polish over top of feather and use brush to press feather onto nail and completely saturate (Figure 12-5).

FIGURE 12-4
While nail is wet, set the feather into the clear polish.

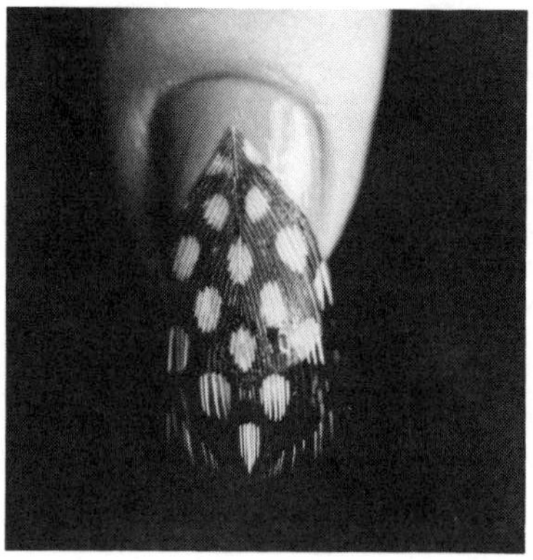

FIGURE 12-5
Apply clear polish over feather and press down with brush.

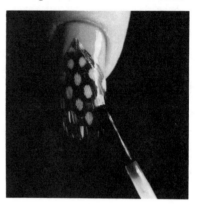

6. Let dry and trim edges of feather as close as possible to nail (Figure 12-6).

7. Complete design with nail gems, tape, or whatever is desired (Figure 12-7).

8. Cover with clear until completely buried in clear polish.

FIGURE 12-6
When dry, trim edges of feather as near to nail as possible.

FIGURE 12-7
Complete design with gems, tapes, or some other choice and cover with clear polish.

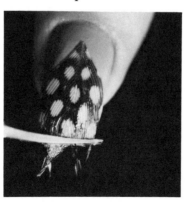
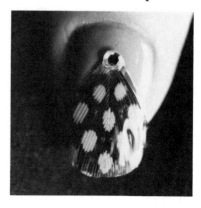

Points to Remember

1. Be sure polish under feather is dry and protected with a dry layer of top coat.
2. Trim feather close to size needed to cover nail portion.
3. Set feather directly on wet top coat and press in place before it dries.
4. After applying polish or other design mediums to nail cover with top coat until it is buried in polish.
5. Apply top coat slowly to avoid bubbles on design.

Gold Leaf Application

This is a very delicate medium to work with. The layers of gold are so thin that they are lighter than a feather. They stick to everything; even things that are not sticky can stick to the thin layers of gold leaf. While working with gold leaf makes, keep tools clean constantly to maintain more control. Do not breathe hard in its direction or it will blow away.

A little speck in the corner of a nail suits some people. Those who prefer a more ornate design can have gold and gems covering part of a feather. Whichever is desired, gold leaf is a popular medium for decoration.

Procedure for Gold Leaf Application

1. Take out the following supplies:

   Orangewood stick   Gold leaf
   Top coat   Tweezers

2. Prepare nail by completing design in gold; then cover with clear polish and let dry.
3. Apply clear nail polish to area for gold design.
4. Use an orangewood stick and tweezers to place bits of gold on nail and press gently into wet polish. If you want more of a solid gold look apply more gold with clear polish.
5. Seal the gold with clear polish. Let dry and, if desired, add to or complete design with tape and/or gems.

Points to Remember

1. Keep tweezers and an orangewood stick clean by wiping polish off constantly. This helps to keep the leaf from sticking to the stick.
2. Use extra polish on the brush when covering gold leaf so it won't stick to the brush.
3. Apply slowly to avoid air bubbles.

Pierced Nail Charm

Pierced is the objective here. Yes, a hole is drilled through the free edge of a nail and a nail charm of choice (there are many to choose from) is bolted onto the nail. Usually real gold is used to make charms with a screw on one side and a bolt in back to hold it in place on the nail. Remarkable as it seems it has been going on for some time and can be very costly depending on the type of charm your client wants. This is a great retail item to carry.

Charms can be put on natural nails that are very strong, but even then, some type of wrap is recommended to support the charm. The hole won't be such a threat to the nail and will be less likely to break.

Procedure for Applying Pierced Nail Charm

1. Take out the following supplies:

   Nail charm
   Charm tool (hand drill for charm, as in Figure 12-8)

FIGURE 12-8
Supplies needed for applying a pierced nail charm.

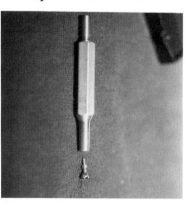

NOTE

Most charm makers hand drills have the bolt wrench built in one end. You should use the drill required for the charm for best results and ease. Remove drill from inside and turn over; reinsert to make handle (see Figures 12-9 through 12-11).

FIGURE 12-9
Remove drill from inside and turn over.

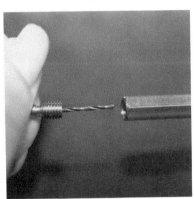

FIGURE 12-10
Reinsert other end into the same hole to make a handle.

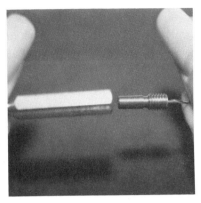

FIGURE 12-11
Drill is ready to use.

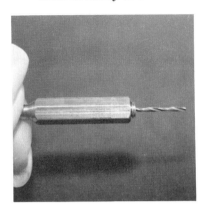

2. Design nail as you want or polish desired color and let nail dry completely.

3. After nail is dry, choose the position of charm. When choosing a place, try not to get too close to the breaking point or the nail might weaken and break. Do not put it too close to the edge or end of nail because the weight of it might weaken it or it can get caught in hair or clothes easily.

4. Support the free edge by placing it on the table firmly. Place drill bit on the spot to be drilled and twist drill clockwise while pressing down on the nail; keep turning and firmly pressing until drill bit has broken through to the other side of nail making a hole to place charm in. Another way to hold the nail is upside down and drill from the back. It is more difficult to be sure you are in the right spot from the back, so doublecheck before you drill the hole.

5. Dust area and clean the nail. Unbolt the back of charm leaving the bolt in the wrench hole (Figure 12-12) and set on its sides so it won't fall out. This keeps you from having to handle the tiny thing and losing it (Figure 12-13).

FIGURE 12-12
Unbolt back of charm.

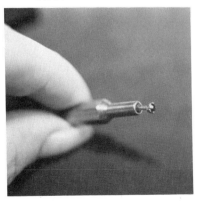

FIGURE 12-13
Leave bolt in wrench hole.

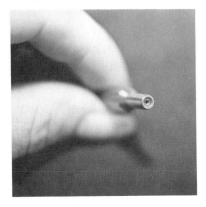

6. Take charm and place it in the hole turning it to the position you want.

7. Take end of drill with bolt in it and put it on the screw. Turn hand a little so you can see that you are putting it on straight. Turn clockwise to tighten bolt to the back of nail.

8. Look at charm to see if it is turned in the right position. If not, slightly loosen the bolt and turn charm to desired position. Try a few different positions to see which is best liked.

9. Once in position tighten bolt while making sure the charm remains in the same position. Sometimes when tightening the bolt the charm moves; so holding it in place is needed.

10. Once the charm is in place and the bolt is properly in place, use clear nail polish to coat the back of the screw and the bolt to prevent it from turning. Apply one coat on top of nail around charm to seal it and keep it from turning. If you polish the nail and cover the charm, you must remove the polish with polish remover. A solid gold nail charm will stand up to acetone but a gold plated one will fade and wear needing to be replaced.

11. If the screw stem on the back of the nail is sticking out too far, cut it off with strong nippers. Some nail charm dealers sell this special tool and other nail charm accessories.

Points to Remember

1. Choose a place for the charm that doesn't look like an easy place to break.

2. Drill a hole straight or the charm will be crooked and not fit flat against the nail.

3. Nail polish must be completely dry or it will mess up when you adjust the charm.

4. Put clear polish on both back and front of the charm to secure it.

5. Don't put clear polish over a gold-plated charm or the gold will rub off when you remove the polish from the charm.

6. If screw stem is sticking out past the back of the nail, cut off the extra part.

Maintaining and Changing Pierced Nail Charms

Soften the clear polish with polish remover and remove the charm carefully with a charm tool. Clean charm with remover and put in safe place until ready to use it again. Remove nail polish and give required service. Polish nails and put the same or a different nail charm in the same hole.

Points to Remember

1. When removing bolt and charm be sure clear polish is melted enough that the charm bolt turns easily.
2. Let polish dry completely before putting a charm on again.

Moving the Charm to a New Place

With nail growth the charm changes places and might need to be moved back or to another nail if wanted. In any case the old hole must be plugged. Plug the hole by using the type of wrap already used on the nail. If supplies are not available to match the wrap, then fill with glue and powder. Cotton can be stuffed into hole and glued and then buffed. Check that both sides of the repaired hole is smooth. Go on to the next service; then apply charm to new place starting over.

Points to Remember

1. Fill the old hole. Don't just cover it up or it will be a weak spot, sure to break or starting cracking.
2. Check that back of nail is smooth where repaired hole is to prevent snagging.

CHAPTER 13

Client Home Care

INTRODUCTION

After all the time and energy spent creating perfectly beautiful nails—no matter how simple or complex the work—in order to protect and prolong your work the client must know how to do that.

Don't be afraid they will run off to do their own nails if you give them too much information about how to care for their nails after they leave the sanctuary of your table.

Tell them how to care for their nails, not how to do them; there is a difference. By giving them this information your work will last longer and in return your clients will be pleased.

Use the following as a guide to the help you can give.

Nail Saver Rules

All clients should be told these nail saver rules for self-care between appointments.

1. To remove or change nail polish while wearing wraps or extensions, the client must use non-acetone nail polish remover to avoid damaging nails.
2. Do not pick at nails to avoid loosening or lifting.

3. Get regular manicures, maintenance service, and fill-in's.

4. If product lifts away from nail and is partially attached, it can be glued only after it is positively clean and dry.

5. Client should obtain home-care supplies. (You can sell your own kits.)

6. If a client glues a broken nail ask them to come in at least to let you check if it will last until the next appointment. This helps avoid a chance of mold or fungus from growing from client's repair.

7. A client with a wrap or extensions should know how to use regular nail polish remover or other proper nail remover to soak nail product off—not to pick or tear at it—to remove it.

Freshen It Up

These are a few simple ways a client can freshen up the polish between appointments.

1. After a few days if nail polish looks dull and scratched one coat of clear polish can renew the shine.

2. If the color chips or gets a deep scratch, another coat of color can cover up the flaws. Seal it with a coat of clear polish.

3. If cuticles start to look dry or ragged, a good cuticle cream rubbed onto cuticles will help.

4. A small buffer used on the edge of the free edge will give a natural nail a clean edge.

Nail Protection Techniques

The techniques listed here can save nails by helping to prevent nail accidents. Information on care is given also.

1. Reaching for anything with a stiff hand or stiff, stretched fingers puts nails in a number one position for disaster. Keep hands and fingers soft and limp until an item is clutched in the hand, not in the fingertips or nails.

2. Removing small items from tabletops or counters can be done by sliding it to the edge and off into the other hand. If there is an edge or lip preventing the slide-off technique, then slide a business card or piece of paper under an item to lift it. It is easy to find something to use if you try.

3. When using the phone, push the buttons with the eraser end of a pencil or any other similar object at hand. If there is nothing to be found then bend your first finger in and press the buttons with your knuckle. This can be done with rotary phones but is more difficult. Other useful items are the end of brushes, lip or eye pencil, hair clip, or whatever is available.

4. To open a door or to lift a car door handle bend the first finger in and use the area from the first knuckle to the second knuckle. That section of the finger can get under the handle and lift it up. Never stick fingers under handle and pull; if you slip, your nails can all snap off backward.

5. Other things to be pulled open should first be grabbed by slowly sliding fingertips through handle and holding on firmly to pull.

6. Use a strong metal or wood object for a tool instead of a fingernail. A quarter or a key can open a flip-top can.

7. Letter openers work better than fingernails.

8. Scissors open packages in the kitchen much quicker and more easily than picking and prying with your nails.

9. Protect your hands and nails from chemicals; if you use them wear rubber gloves.

10. If doing any messy craft work, protect nails with work gloves.

11. To fasten a button, hold the button with the side of first finger and the outer edge of thumb instead of fingertips. Holding the button by the edge of fingers keeps the button from sliding under the fingernail and making it difficult to button.

12. When pulling clothes on, grab on tightly with the thumb and second knuckle of the first finger and then pull. If you pull when holding on with fingertips garment can slip easily and get caught on nails and may break or damage one or several nails.

Client Home-Care Kits

The client home-care kit can be made by you and sold to every client for a profit. It also will enable them to maintain proper nail care between appointments. If you do not want retail profits, provide a list of necessary items.

Suggested Kit Contents

The following items can be provided by you or listed as necessary to ensure proper self-care nail maintenance.

1. Clear top coat nail polish
2. Bottle of nail polish (client's choice)
3. Small nail buffer
4. Nail glue
5. Nail sanitation solution
6. Cuticle cream or hand cream
7. Short orangewood stick
8. Non-acetone nail polish remover
9. Small nail remover solution
10. Several business cards

Client Home Repair Instructions

If a client damages or breaks a nail, it can be an untimely disaster. Not knowing what to do can make it worse. Ease the mind of your client by explaining what can be done to keep it together and quickly fix that nail at least to hold it until they can come in for a repair. It is best to know how to quickly and easily glue it back together the right way instead of guessing and making a mess. Your clients will love you for showing them how to get out of a nail jam without you. As dependent as all clients become you can't always be there to glue a crack. Every client should have a home-care kit or the items listed for an emergency repair job. Directions for how to fix a lifting wrap, how to glue a broken nail, and how to fix a cracked nail are given below.

Fix a Lifting Wrap

1. Be sure nail is completely dry.
2. Gently press the end of the nail to expose the lifting wrap.
3. Holding the end, put a little drop of glue at the very edge of the wrap and let the glue slide under it. Quickly press the underside of free edge up, which in return will make the wrap press down into the glue. Wipe away any extra glue before it dries.
4. Come into the salon as soon as possible to get it checked and get the required attention.

Glue a Broken Nail

1. Hold the broken end of the nail to the breaking place on the nail and match it to see if it will fit together. Most of the time a nail can be put together like a puzzle piece.
2. Apply glue evenly on the breaking point end and place the piece of nail right up next to it. Line it up perfectly before touching them together.
3. Once in place hold for five or ten seconds depending on type of glue used (fast- or slow-drying).
4. Wipe extra glue from the top of nail and clean under the free edge.
5. Go to salon and get it fixed.

Fix a Cracked Nail

1. Put glue on backside of nail and let it dry. A second coat can be used for more strength.
2. Go to the salon as soon as possible to have the nail fixed correctly. The only way to fix a crack is to remove the wrap, repair the crack, and then wrap it again.

<u>NOTE</u>

All home repairs should be sanitized if possible
and checked soon by a professional. Clients must know
this is a temporary solution until the nail can
get fixed properly.

CHAPTER 14

Your Business

INTRODUCTION

How far you go in the nail business depends on you. There really is no limit, no rule that says you have to stop at any point. You can start working for someone in their salon and before you know it you can own one or more salons. Some nail technicians have even gone as far as to develop their own line of nail products or to develop a special technique they can teach to others for a profit. Or, like me, after ten years of doing nails and teaching nail artistry in New York you can write a book.
If you have the desire to be successful you can go as far as you want in the field of advanced nail techniques.

Money Making Options

There are several ways to utilize your nail care skills. Listed are three of the most used options. No matter which option you choose have business cards made up to promote yourself wherever you work.

1. Work in a beauty or nail salon for a salary or commission.
2. Rent a space for your table in a salon.
3. Start your own nail salon.

When choosing which option is best for you, consider how much experience you have. You wouldn't want to open your own salon until you are quite good and have experienced the many different situations that can arise in the nail business. With experience and knowledge of how a salon operates you have a better chance of having your own successful nail salon. Each of the three different options are explained in detail.

Salons and Salary or Commission

When you get a job in a salon you usually must go along with whatever method of payment is in use. Some salons start you on a salary or hourly rate. To receive a commission you must bring in receipts that are over your regular salary by a predetermined amount. Usually it is double what you make. Any amount over double your normal salary determines your commission. To make it simple, you either get your salary or your commission, whichever is greater. If you do not make more in commissions than your regular salary, then you will get at least your salary. This protects you so that you will always get at the least a regular paycheck no less than the regular salary including your tips. Base salary and commission rate should be predetermined before you start.

Some salons prefer to pay a straight salary or a straight commission. In this case, you should get either a higher base salary or a higher commission than you normally would on a salary against commission basis. Check into company benefits. Some large salon chains offer great benefits to employees.

Renting a Space in a Salon

This is a very popular way of setting up business. Find a salon that is willing to rent you space for your table and storage for supplies. You can have your own business with very little overhead. Work out the details of what you need from the salon and what the salon expects from you before you determine the rental rate. A written agreement will help avoid any misunderstandings. The following is a list of questions to be answered before you rent a space.

1. How much room do you get?
2. Can you use window space for advertisement?
3. How much locked storage space is available?
4. Can you retail your own nail products?

5. Is there room for you to expand by getting another table and hiring your own employee to do nails?

6. Are utilities, phone, receptionist and any other part of the salon available for your use?

When you are in this type of business situation other business facts that must be addressed include insurance, business certificates, and health department certificates.

Insurance, Business Certificates, and Health Department Certificates

Insurance is a must. You need to find out if you are covered under the salon policy, if you can be added on to it, or if you have to cover yourself separately. Laws differ from state to state and need to be checked; you do not want to be put out of business because of one mishappening. It is equally important to check your taxes and abide them; be sure also to check into business certificates and health department regulations. You may be covered under the salon's business and health certificates; or, if you are considered a separate business, you may need your own. A lease for term of rental time can protect you from being evicted after the owner sees the profits they are missing by not having their own nail services.

Overhead

Your overhead for doing nails depends on the money making option you choose. When working in a salon on a salary or commission the salon usually supplies the products needed. If you prefer particular products that are unavailable you have to get them yourself. A fair employer will repay you for it.

If you are on a very high straight commission you might be required to supply all of your own products.

If you are renting space in a salon you must supply everything as well as pay rent for your space. You need to have enough business to cover the expenses. That is why it is best to start out working for someone until you build a following—that is, clients who will follow you wherever you go to work. When you decide to start your own business they will follow you, which gives you a better starting advantage.

To open your own salon is of course the most costly. You are paying rent and other bills, as well as paying for supplies to do the nail services.

Potential Profits

To say how much money you can expect to make is not really possible. Every nail technician works differently. The determining factor is how many clients can be done in one day and what services are offered. If it takes you one hour to extend and wrap ten fingernails and you charge $50 or if it takes you a half-hour to do a manicure that cost $10, then you can see that one extension with wraps is more profitable then two manicures. You have to give manicures so you need to raise the price and do it very specially or perfect your techniques so you can do great manicures in fifteen minutes.

If you are in business for yourself then you get profits from one or more employees. The more employees and clients you have, the more money is made.

For example, in one day you could do four sets of nails at $50 each and two maintenance manicures at $15 each, two fill-ins at $20 each, and a manicure at $10. That is $280 in one day. If you have similar days, five days a week, you gross $1400 a week or $4800 a month, depending on the appointment book.

If you work in a salon for commission at 50 percent, you would make $140 plus tips in one day. If you are renting you keep all of it but you take rent and supply costs out. If you own a salon, you pay employees and other costs.

It all really depends on your personal abilities.

Owning Your Own Shop

This can be wonderful as well as financially rewarding. Remember, however, you must be financially prepared to run a business especially one that is just starting out. Be sure you can cover overhead expenses until you have established a steady clientele and are making a profit. When you are a salon owner, you are responsible for everything. Decide if you are capable of not only working, but also of running the whole business all at the same time. Otherwise, you may want to consider getting professional help with the management. Be sure to get proper legal and financial assistance prior to starting. If you have never been in business for yourself it might be wise to take a small business course to learn "How to run a business."

Choosing Your Location, Things to Consider

The following questions only outline things to consider. Many more may arise as you plan and set up your business.

Is it a busy area?

Can a sign be easily seen from the street?

Is it easy to find?

Is there good parking?

How long is the lease?

Is there room to expand?

How much is the rent?

Is there an option to buy?

Things You Need to Get Started

Some basic services and equipment needs to determine prior to setting up a salon include:

Appointment book

Good receptionist

Trained professional employees

Product for salon use

Retail products

Business cards

Appointment cards

Advertisement

Proper licensing (according to your state law)

Recommended tax accountant

First and last months' rent

Electric

Telephone

Water

Interior of salon (workstation, front desk, lounge)

Extra startup fees, hidden cost

Retail Profits

To boost your profits from the nail business you can sell retail nail-care items to clients for use at home. Some clients like to freshen their polish or change it themselves. Sell them the color they wear along with base and top coats. Also home-repair supplies or kits can be put together by you. If you supply your clients with items your clients use and if they are going to go out and buy them, why not buy them from you?

The following lists suggested items you can buy and re-sell to clients:

1. Nail polish remover for artificial nails
2. Base coat
3. Colored polish
4. Top coat
5. Nail glue
6. Buffer
7. Orangewood stick
8. Corrector sticks
9. Cuticle creams and conditioners
10. Nail art supplies
11. Gold nails or nail jewelry
12. Gift certificates

You can sell items separately or make different kits or sets of supplies tailored to each client's needs.

Determining Price

The facts involved in determining what to charge for each nail service are:

How much experience you have
Quality of your work
How much time it takes for each service
Location of salon
Type of clients

The amount of experience, quality of work and time it takes plus the location of salon equals the price to charge.

If you check the nearby competition as to their prices and the kinds of services they offer, compare it to yours. This will give you a good idea of what to charge.

Suggested Service List

All nail services should be offered if you want to provide the maximum. These include:

Manicure and pedicure
Nail tips and nail biter tips
Cosmetic nail and corrective nail techniques
Linen and silk nail wrapping
Acrylic nails, sculptured and over tips
Fiberglass nail techniques
Ultraviolet gel nails and no light gel nails
Maintenance manicure and fill-ins
Patching nail wraps, cotton patching
Polish change and nail art

Some nail specialists excel at one or two methods and provide only these few but still get a lot of work all the time.

When you find a method that is easy and fast for you and satisfies your clients stick with it. Try to learn all the techniques possible because you can never know too much and you never know when you will need the skill.

Whichever route you choose always keep in mind perfection and do not settle for anything less than best. Don't do any job less than you would want for yourself and keep your standards high.

If you keep a good attitude and let it show through your work, you will do lots of nails and have many happy clients.

Author's Note

Always continue to educate yourself and update your knowledge of new procedures and products that are on the way.

Nail and beauty trade shows really are great, informative, and lots of fun.

Subscribe to trade magazines which can be found at the trade shows. Ask your local beauty school or call your local convention center for dates on trade show events.

(Keep on buffing.)

Tammy Bigan